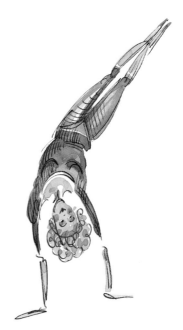

Take Off 10 Years in 10 Weeks

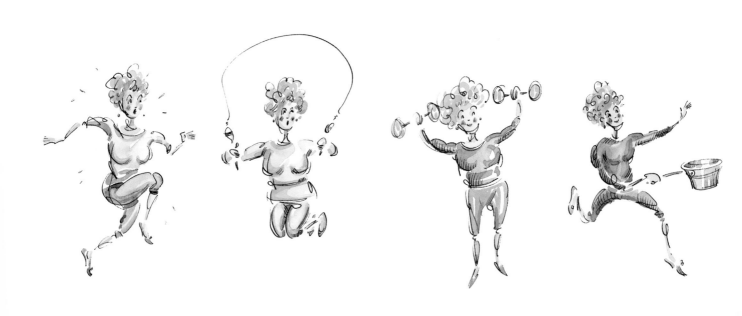

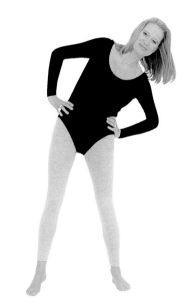

Take Off 10 Years in 10 Weeks

Judith Wills

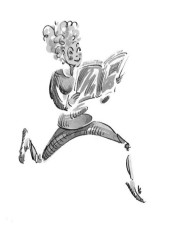

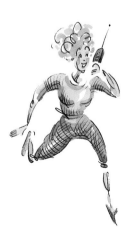

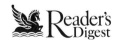

Reader's Digest

THE READER'S DIGEST ASSOCIATION, INC.
Pleasantville, New York/Montreal

To Mother and Ann

A READER'S DIGEST BOOK
Conceived, edited and designed by Quadrille Publishing Ltd

PUBLISHING DIRECTOR: Anne Furniss
ART DIRECTOR: Mary Evans
PROJECT EDITOR: Lewis Esson
DESIGN: Mary Staples
EDITORIAL ASSISTANT: Katherine Seely
SPECIAL PHOTOGRAPHY: Ian Hooton
ILLUSTRATIONS: Lynne Robinson and Julia Whatley
PICTURE REASEARCH: Nadine Bazar
PRODUCTION: Candida Lane

Consultants
WARDROBE STYLING: Ceril Campbell
MAKEUP: Celia Hunter
HAIR DRESSING: Paul Edmonds
EXERCISES: Louise Taylor

Library of Congress Cataloging in Publication Data

Wills, Judith.
Take off 10 years in 10 weeks: a change-your-life program for the outer you, the vital you, and the inner you / Judith Wills.
p. cm.
ISBN 0 89577-899-8
1. Middle-aged women–Health and hygiene.   2.Weight loss.
3.Physical fitness for women 1. Title
RA778.W563 1996
613.7'045–dc20   96-31828

Printed and bound in Spain

The author and publishers would like to stress that this book expresses the well-informed opinions and experience of the author. Although we are confident that almost everyone will benefit from this book, we can in no way guarantee results of any kind. Whether or not you have any pre-existing medical condition, seek your physician's advice and undergo a full physical examination before starting the program.

CONTENTS

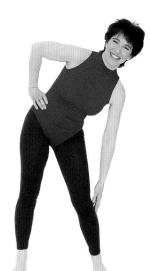

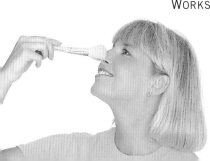

"I'm proud to be my age," said a 45-year-old colleague of mine
when she heard that I was writing this book.
*"Why do you want to encourage women to think they've got
to act and look like 25-year-olds?"* she quite reasonably asked.

Well I don't. This book isn't about mimicking youth. I have no intention of helping you to look, or be, the same as you were then, or, indeed, of asking you to become a carbon copy of your teenage daughter. You don't want that; I don't want that.

But what I do set out to do is *improve* upon youth. To steal its assets, such as vitality and optimism, a fit body and glowing skin, and leave the rest very gladly behind.

I'm proud to say I'm 46. But I still enjoy it when I'm taken for 40, or even less. To me, it means I look after myself and that I care enough about life, and the people I love, to make an effort. And, of course, I very much hope that looking after myself means I will feel healthier and happier into a long and fulfilling old age!

I know what you want, because it is what I want – to be, simply, my best for now. Your best, for now, is what this book is all about. Looking your best, feeling your best and enjoying your life. Why look old, why feel old when you needn't? Why get left behind?

Take Off 10 Years in 10 Weeks is the program that helps get you back on track in every way—maybe, even, to find a new track. All I ask is that you promise to put yourself first, at least some of the time—something that many of you have *not* done in years. Women who have been adults through the 60s, 70s, 80s, or 90s have, I believe, had the hardest, busiest, most stressful time of any generation of women, with choices, responsibilities, and problems that no other women have had to face.

Now is your time.
Time to get back in touch with yourself, your body and your needs.
And here is *your* book.

The 10-week course it contains has been tested by ordinary women aged between 35 and 57. You'll encounter several of them many times in the pages ahead as you work through the program yourself. If you need inspiration or confirmation that you really can shed the years and feel so much better, look at the four participants who appear on the opposite page (as they were at the start of the 10 weeks), then look on page 138, ten weeks later, and read the women's comments, too.

Ten weeks can change your life—if you let them!

Judith Wills

Meet the Participants

*Meet our four main participants, Hilary, Sue, Pamela, and Kay.
You'll be finding out much more about each of them, and how they are progressing,
as you work through the 10-week course.*

Hilary Clarke

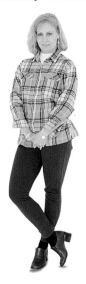

Sue Salkind

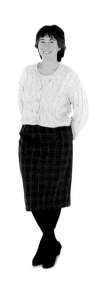

Pamela Newton

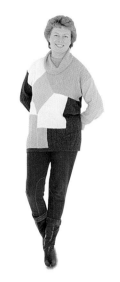

Kay Rainford

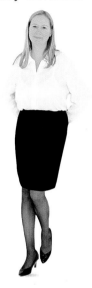

Hilary is a 43-year-old nursery nurse and married with two grown-up sons and a teenage daughter.

She has put on nearly 20 pounds since her 20s and has virtually given up buying new clothes, "because it is depressing when nothing looks right."

A recent two-year college course made the problem worse – "I couldn't resist the desserts in the college café!" and, although she goes to the swimming pool regularly, Hilary has difficulty sometimes in doing even one length. "I get out of breath and feel dreadful – so I really want to get fitter."

Hilary admits she hasn't changed her hairstyle or makeup in several years and is looking for new advice, as well as for some help with her problem skin, her lack of energy and stress levels.

Sue, 39, is a part-time physician, mother of two small daughters and is doing a course in acupuncture. Sue currently weighs about 140 pounds – "Most of which appears to be around my tummy!" – and is finding it difficult to motivate herself to exercise.

"As a doctor, I feel I should set a good example to my patients, but I'm afraid I don't. I am also something of a chocoholic and have got quite lazy in my eating habits. I really need you to give me the motivation I need to shape up and get fitter."

Sue also admits that she is in dire need of a wardrobe re-think. "I've bought hardly anything new since my girls were born and I've no confidence in shopping for myself. And I've never worn makeup, either." I think it's time for a new look Sue. . .

Pamela is 57 and a homemaker. She has two grown-up sons and is a grandmother. She lives with her husband, who is retired, and although she bowls and swims in the summer, two of her favorite hobbies – eating out and entertaining at home – have resulted in a serious weight gain over the years.

"I used to be a very slim 35-23-35, and it really depresses me when I catch a glimpse of myself unexpectedly. I love nice clothes but nothing looks good on me any more."

Pamela is on hormone replacement therapy and feels this is going to stop her losing weight. "I don't want to give up my life style, either. I wonder what you are going to be able to do to help *me*!"

Kay, 49, is suffering a total loss of confidence, having lost her job as an administration assistant two years agoand having been rejected for hundreds of other posts. "I feel my age is against me when applying for jobs," she says. "I think it would really help me to get somewhere if I look younger and feel better." She is also recently divorced and living alone for the first time in her life.

At 140 pounds, Kay, who is also on hormone replacement therapy after a hysterectomy the same year as her divorce and losing her job ("not a great year, really!"), is hardly overweight but she has never done any exercise and her body really is badly out of condition. "I'm stuck in a time-warp as far as hair and clothes go, too. I feel the need of a complete overhaul!"

*You will also be meeting Sal, Linda, and Angela during the program, each of whom also
completed the 10-week course with our four participants above.*

YOUR 10-WEEK TIMETABLE

Your schedule for the 10-week course begins opposite.
First read the notes below.

THE COURSE IS DIVIDED INTO THREE SECTIONS. THESE ARE:

MIRROR IMAGE
The Outer You,

which deals with your body size and shape,
your skin, makeup, hair, and wardrobe.

ENERGY SOURCES
The Vital You,

which enhances and taps into your energy levels
in every possible way.

LIFE CHOICES
The Inner You,

which helps you to explore possibilities and
rethink your life.

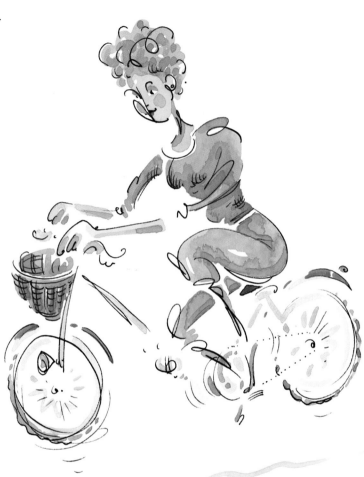

*Beginning of
Week*

1

_____
weight

_____
bust

_____
waist

_____
hips

_____
thighs

_____
BMI ★

_____
WHR ★

_____
energy levels

COMMENTS

E ach of the three sections is divided into workshops, which we will be covering during the next 10 weeks. Some workshops, such as your eating plan and the ShapeWise programs, are ongoing throughout the 10 weeks and beyond. Others are short "lessons" or assessments, which may take between 20 and 60 minutes of your time. I aim for the weekly time input on the course to be no more than three hours a week, plus occasional "specials."

All you need to do is follow the week-by-week timetable as it is laid out in the next 10 pages. Before you begin, read the introductions to each

of the three sections (Mirror Image on page 19, Energy Sources on page 93, and Life Choices on page 118), which will give you a clear idea of what we're planning to achieve.

At the start of each week, look at the workshops you're going to be covering in the week ahead, and schedule them into your week, using your own calendar. For your own personal record, fill in all the blank weight, statistics, energy levels and comment boxes as you go along.

Also, have a photo taken as you are now, then take one at the end of the 10 weeks just like our participants did.

★ *see page 21*

_____
weight

_____
bust

_____
waist

_____
hips

_____
thighs

_____
energy levels

COMMENTS

General notes:

- Fill in your weight and other statistics opposite.

- Look at what we'll be doing in the week ahead and the time
it may take, and plan your own schedule accordingly.

- Do the Assessments as early in the week as possible.

- Plan the most demanding workshops for your least busy days.

- Your personal eating plan will be ongoing through the weeks–take time
to plan your menus and to shop.

- Leave at least one day between each ShapeWise session
to allow your body to recover.

WEEK ONE SCHEDULE

workshop		page	time	notes
	Mirror Image			
I	**SIZING-UP** – BODYWISE ASSESSMENT	20	*45 min.*	
2	**PERSONAL EATING PLAN**	24	*Ongoing*	*Read through and familiarize.*
3	**SHAPEWISE 1** – TOTAL TONE Session 1	36	*30 min.*	*Familiarize.*
3	**SHAPEWISE 1** – TOTAL TONE Session 2	36	*20 min.*	*Your first real workout!*
3	**SHAPEWISE 1** – TOTAL TONE Session 3	36	*20 min.*	
	Energy Sources			
II	**HEALTH CHECK**	94	*45 min.*	*Make appointments as necessary.*
I2	**TIME MANAGEMENT**	96	*30 min.*	*Time allowed includes keeping daily diary.*
	Life Choices			
I8	**NETWORKING**	119	*30 min.*	*Read through; decide what is relevant to you; make a plan.*

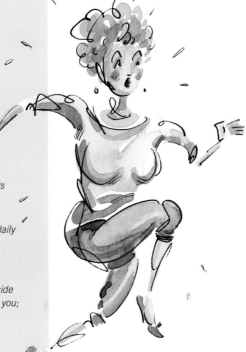

End of Week

2

_____
weight

_____
bust

_____
waist

_____
hips

_____
thighs

_____
energy levels

COMMENTS
_____

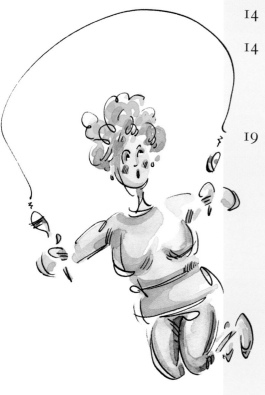

WEEK TWO SCHEDULE

workshop		page	time	notes
Mirror Image				
2	**PERSONAL EATING PLAN**	24	Ongoing	
3	**SHAPEWISE** – TOTAL TONE Session 1	36	*20 min.*	
3	**SHAPEWISE** – TOTAL TONE Session 2	36	*20 min.*	
3	**SHAPEWISE** – TOTAL TONE Session 3	36	*20 min.*	
5	**BARE ESSENTIALS**	52	*20 min.*	*Read through.*
5	**BARE ESSENTIALS**	52	*15 min.*	*Shop for items needed when convenient.*
Energy Sources				
12	**TIME MANAGEMENT**	96	*20 min.*	*Analyze your week 1 daily diary using guidelines in workshop. Write down your intentions. How much time can you save?*
14	**IMPROVE YOUR STAMINA**	105	*30 min.*	*Read through and do the Measured Mile Test.*
14	**IMPROVE YOUR STAMINA**	105	*20 min.*	*Start on Stage 1.*
Life Choices				
19	**EDUCATION**	122	*45 min.*	*Read through; make your own plans.*

WEEK THREE SCHEDULE

workshop		page	time	notes
	Mirror Image			
2	**PERSONAL EATING PLAN**	24	*Ongoing*	
3	**SHAPEWISE 1** – TOTAL TONE Session 1	36	*20 min.*	
3	**SHAPEWISE 1** – TOTAL TONE Session 2	36	*20 min.*	
3	**SHAPEWISE 1** – TOTAL TONE Session 3	36	*20. min.*	
4	**SHAPEWISE 2** – BODY ALIGNMENT	48	*20 min.*	*Read through and do Mirror Test. Familiarize yourself with exercises.*
5	**BARE ESSENTIALS** – 20-Minute Facial	56	*20 min.*	*Ideal time for this is after a bath.*
	Energy Sources			
14	**STAMINA** – Session 1	105	*20 min.*	
14	**STAMINA** – Session 2	105	*20 min.*	
14	**STAMINA** – Mind Games	107	*15 min.*	*Try this as often as you like.*
	Life Choices			
20	**EXPLORATION**	124	*20 min.*	

_____

weight

_____

bust

_____

waist

_____

hips

_____

thighs

_____

energy levels

COMMENTS

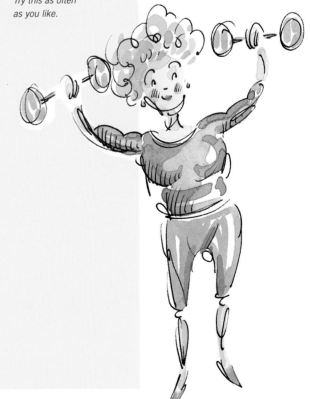

End of Week

4

weight

bust

waist

hips

thighs

energy levels

COMMENTS

WEEK FOUR SCHEDULE

	workshop	page	time	notes
	Mirror Image			
2	**PERSONAL EATING PLAN**	24	*Ongoing*	
3	**SHAPEWISE 1**– TOTAL TONE Session 1	36	*20 min.*	
3	**SHAPEWISE 1**– TOTAL TONE Session 2	36	*20 min.*	
3	**SHAPEWISE 1**– TOTAL TONE Session 3	36	*20 min.*	
4	**SHAPEWISE 2** – BODY ALIGNMENT	48	*5 min.*	*Optional.*
5	**BARE ESSENTIALS** – Surgery-Free Face-Lift	55	*15 min.*	*Try to do these exercises for 2-3 minutes twice a day through the program.*
	Energy Sources			
14	**STAMINA** Session 1	105	*20 min.*	
14	**STAMINA** Session 2	105	*20 min.*	
14	**STAMINA** Session 3	105	*20 min.*	
15	**LEARN TO RELAX**	108	*30 min.*	*Read through and put into context of your own life.*
	Life Choices			
21	**SOCIABILITY** – FRIENDS	126	*15 min.*	

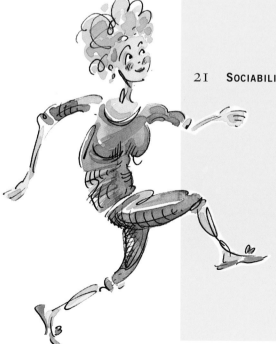

WEEK FIVE SCHEDULE

workshops	page	time	notes

Mirror Image

		page	time	notes
2	**PERSONAL EATING PLAN**	24	*Ongoing*	
3	**SHAPEWISE 1**– TOTAL TONE Session 1	36	*20 min.*	
3	**SHAPEWISE 1** – TOTAL TONE Session 2	36	*20 min.*	
3	**SHAPEWISE 1** – TOTAL TONE Session 3	36	*20 min.*	
4	**SHAPEWISE 2** – BODY ALIGNMENT	48	*5 min.*	*Optional.*
6	**MAKEUP MAGIC**	58	*30 min.*	*Read through and study photos and ideas.*

Energy Sources

14	**STAMINA** – Session 1	105	*20 min.*
14	**STAMINA** – Session 2	105	*20 min.*
14	**STAMINA** – Session 3	105	*20 min.*
15	**LEARN TO RELAX** – SELF-MASSAGE	110	*10 min.*

Life Choices

21	**SOCIABILITY** – FAMILY MATTERS	129	*30 min.*

weight

bust

waist

hips

thighs

energy levels

COMMENTS

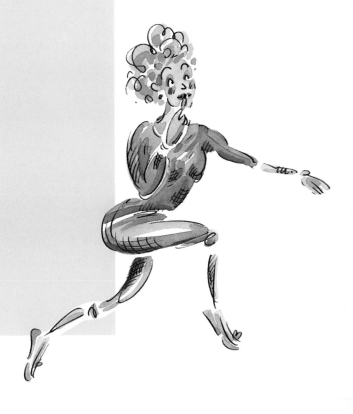

End of Week

6

weight
_____

bust
_____

waist
_____

hips
_____

thighs
_____

energy levels
_____

COMMENTS
_____

WEEK SIX SCHEDULE

workshop		page	time	notes
	Mirror Image			
2	**PERSONAL EATING PLAN**	24	*Ongoing*	
3	**SHAPEWISE 1** – TOTAL TONE Session 1	36	*20 min.*	
3	**SHAPEWISE 1** – TOTAL TONE Session 2	36	*20 min.*	
3	**SHAPEWISE 1** – TOTAL TONE Session 3	36	*20 min.*	
4	**SHAPEWISE 2** – BODY ALIGNMENT	48	*5 min.*	*Optional.*
6	**MAKEUP MAGIC**	58	*1 hour*	*Go through your own make-up and decide what you need to throw away or buy. Buy what you need, taking advantage of store make-overs.*
	Energy Sources			
14	**STAMINA** – Session 1	105	*20 min.+*	*Increase your time when ready.*
14	**STAMINA** – Session 2	105	*20 min.+*	
14	**STAMINA** – Session 3	105	*20 min.+*	
16	**DEEP SLEEP**	112	*15 min.*	*Optional for insomnia. Read through and see what you would like to try.*
	Life Choices			
22	**RELATIONSHIPS 1**	130	*30 min.*	*For women already in a relationship.*
or				
23	**RELATIONSHIPS 2**	132	*30 min.*	*For women seeking a relationship.*

WEEK SEVEN SCHEDULE

	workshop	page	time	notes
	Mirror Image			
2	**Personal Eating Plan**	24	*Ongoing*	Don't forget–once you reach target weight, move to the Zest Plan on page 103.
3	**Shapewise 1** – Total Tone Session 1	36	*20 min.*	
3	**Shapewise 1** – Total Tone Session 2	36	*20 min.*	
3	**Shapewise 1** – Total Tone Session 3	36	*20 min.*	
4	**Shapewise 2** – Body Alignment	48	*5 min.*	Optional – if you have poor posture you will benefit from daily Shapewise 2 sessions.
6	**Makeup Magic**	58	*20 min.*	Give yourself a new makeup look using your new cosmetics, and the information in the workshop for guidance.
7	**Hair Flair 1** – Superstyles	66	*20 min.+*	
	Energy Sources			
14	**Stamina** – Session 1	105	*20 min.+*	
14	**Stamina** – Session 2	105	*20 min.+*	
14	**Stamina** – Session 3	105	*20 min.+*	
17	**Zapping the Negatives**	115	*20 min.*	
	Life Choices			
24	**Pure Pleasure**	136	*20 min.*	

weight

bust

waist

hips

thighs

energy levels

Comments

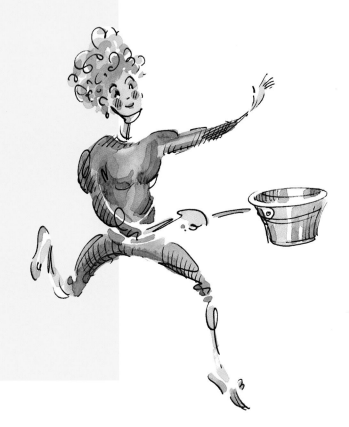

End of Week

8

weight
_____

bust
_____

waist
_____

hips
_____

thighs
_____

energy levels

COMMENTS
_____

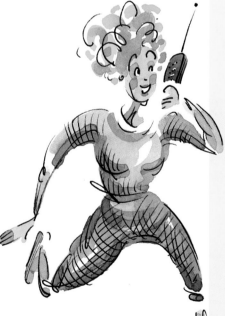

WEEK EIGHT SCHEDULE

workshop		page	time	notes

Mirror Image

	workshop	page	time	notes
2	**PERSONAL EATING PLAN**	24	*Ongoing*	
3	**SHAPEWISE 1** – TOTAL TONE Session 1	36	*20 min.*	
3	**SHAPEWISE 1** – TOTAL TONE Session 2	36	*20 min.*	
3	**SHAPEWISE 1** – TOTAL TONE Session 3	36	*20 min.*	
4	**SHAPEWISE 2** – BODY ALIGNMENT	48	*5 min.*	*Optional.*
7	**HAIR FLAIR 1** – SUPERSTYLES	66	*1 hour+*	*Get hair styled using notes on page 69 to help you and stylist achieve the look you want.*
8	**HAIR FLAIR 2** – COLOR AND CONDITION	70	*15 min.*	*Read through the workshop and think about what you'd like to achieve.*
9	**STYLE ASSESSMENT 1** – FINDING YOUR OWN STYLE	76	*20 min.+*	

Energy Sources

	workshop	page	time	notes
14	**STAMINA** – Session 1	105	*20 min.+*	
14	**STAMINA** – Session 2	105	*20 min.+*	
14	**STAMINA** – Session 3	105	*20 min.+*	
12	**TIME MANAGEMENT**	96		
15	**LEARN TO RELAX**	108	*30 min.*	*Reread these four workshops; assess your own progress; make notes for future.*
16	**DEEP SLEEP**	112		
17	**ZAPPING THE NEGATIVES**	115		

Life Choices

	workshop	page	time	notes
18	**NETWORKING**	119	*20 min*	*Check how your plans for both workshops are progressing.*
19	**EDUCATION**	122	*20 min*	

WEEK NINE SCHEDULE

	workshop	page	time	notes
	Mirror Image			
2	**Personal Eating Plan**	24	*Ongoing*	
3	**Shapewise 1** – Total Tone Session 1	36	*20 min.*	
3	**Shapewise 1** – Total Tone Session 2	36	*20 min.*	
3	**Shapewise 1** – Total Tone Session 3	36	*20 min.*	
4	**Shapewise 2** – Body Alignment	48	*5 min.*	*Optional*
9	**Style Assessment 1** – Wardrobe Workout	85	*1 hour*	*Sort out your wardrobe following the guidelines in part of the box on page 85.*
10	**Style Assessment 2** – Dressing for Your Shape	86	*1 hour*	*Read the workshop and assess your pared-down wardrobe for "shape suitability." Decide what, if anything, you need to buy.*
	Energy Sources			
14	**Stamina** – Session 1	105	*20 min.+*	
14	**Stamina** – Session 2	105	*20 min.+*	
14	**Stamina** – Session 3	105	*20 min.+*	
	Life Choices			
20	**Exploration**	124	*20 min.*	*Reread these two workshops and assess your own progress. Make notes for the future.*
21	**Sociability**	126	*20 min.*	

weight

bust

waist

hips

thighs

energy levels

COMMENTS

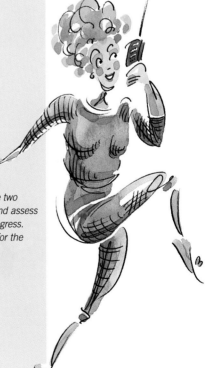

End of Week

10

weight
_____

bust
_____

waist
_____

hips
_____

thighs
_____

BMI ★
_____

WHR ★
_____

energy levels
_____

COMMENTS

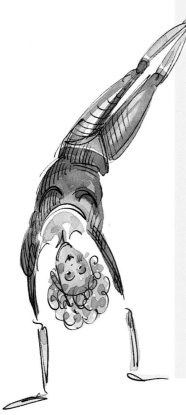

WEEK TEN SCHEDULE

	workshop	page	time	notes
	Mirror Image			
I	**BODY ASSESSMENTS**	20	*15 min.*	*Reassess your BMI, WHR, your target weight, and your shape; write your comments.*
2	**PERSONAL EATING PLAN**	24	*Ongoing*	
3	**SHAPEWISE 1** – TOTAL TONE Session 1	36	*20 min.*	
3	**SHAPEWISE 1** – TOTAL TONE Session 2	36	*20 min.*	
3	**SHAPEWISE 1** – TOTAL TONE Session 3	36	*20 min.*	
4	**SHAPEWISE 2** – BODY ALIGNMENT	48	*5 min.*	*Optional.*
8	**HAIR FLAIR 2** – COLOR AND CONDITION	70	*1-2 hours*	*Optional. If you're not sure about changing color, ask the head colorist at your salon.*
9	**STYLE ASSESSMENT 1** – SHOPPING TRIP	85	*half day+*	*Choose some new clothes; you deserve them.*

	Energy Sources			
II	**HEALTH CHECK**	94	*1 hour*	
14	**STAMINA** – SESSION 1	105	*20 min.+*	
14	**STAMINA** – SESSION 2	105	*20 min.+*	
14	**STAMINA** – SESSION 3	105	*20 min.+*	

	Life Choices			
22	**RELATIONSHIPS 1**	130		
	or		*20 min.*	*Re-read these two workshops and note the improvements you've made.*
23	**RELATIONSHIPS 2**	132		
24	**PURE PLEASURE**	136		

Congratulations!

You have completed the 10-week course. Check out your final weight and statistics; assess how you feel.

Take that photo of yourself with your new hair and makeup, wearing some new clothes and a big smile.

Compare it with how you looked 10 weeks ago; how you looked 10 years ago.

Please write and let me know your verdict and send me those photos!

★ see page 21

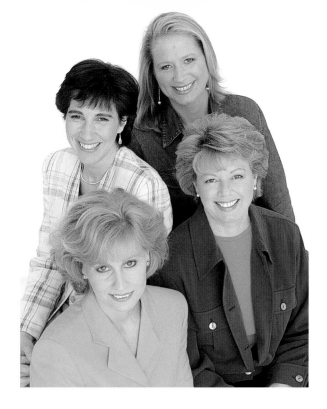

MIRROR IMAGE
The Outer You

How long since you took a good look in the mirror? How long since you liked what you saw? In fact, how long since you noticed how you really look? It can become very easy to get used to extra pounds or inches; flabbiness where your flesh used to be firm. "I'm getting older–I might as well accept it" goes the familiar cry.

No. No, no, NO! The Mirror Image workshops will help you to see yourself afresh and to make objective decisions about what you can change, what those changes should be, and how to go about them. It is *never* too late to restyle your body and your looks and shed the years. Your body doesn't have to succumb to middle-aged spread.

Research reveals that exercise in mid-life shows results just as quickly as it did in your 20s. And losing weight, while a slower process than when you were young, is not as impossible a task as you may believe!

In the same way, old familiar hair, makeup, and style looks may be comforting and easy–but it's a very rare woman indeed who can look her best with the same makeup, hair, and wardrobe she had ten–even five–years ago.

Whether you just need updating, or gave up trying to look your best years ago–and now go makeup free, with your hair pulled back, and living in leggings and a baggy sweatshirt–you'll find the answers here. Your body deserves some attention. Now is the time to give it. Here is the place.

*F*ew women approaching–or in–their middle years have a body as slim or as firm as it was in their teens and 20s. In Workshop 1, we will assess your physical appearance and make realistic decisions about just how far you can turn back time.

WORKSHOP **1** SIZING-UP

Your Weight

One of the most common physical signs of aging is weight gain. So many of us experience this that the dreaded "middle-age spread" is thought of as natural and inevitable. The woman of 40 who can still fit into the wedding dress she wore at 20 is seen as something of a phenomenon. And the truth is that to stay as slim as you were in your teens and 20s, you do need to eat less than you did then (you'll find more on the reasons for this in Workshop 2).

However, don't be too envious of those few skinny women, because some of the latest research shows that putting on a little weight as we get older is probably a good thing, and that being thin and living on a meager diet is not. One common consequence of thinness is an increased risk of osteoporosis, which any sensible woman would prefer to avoid. There is also evidence that menopausal symptoms may be more severe in thin women. And, should you–like most of us–fear wrinkles as much as being fat, a thin face is much more likely to show wrinkles than one "plumped up" by a thin layer of fat.

No, what you want to achieve is *balance*–a weight that is, perhaps, up to 15 pounds heavier than that which you were at 20 (if you were slim then), but not much more. Too much fat is aging and even worse for your health than being too thin. A good rule of thumb for how much weight gain is acceptable for you is to put on no more than three to four pounds for every decade you are over 25. So if

Can I lose weight if I'm on Hormone Replacement Therapy (HRT)?

If you are overweight and on HRT – yes, you can lose weight. There is no scientific evidence that shows you have to gain weight with HRT–though many women do. And, as our participants Kay and Pamela, both on HRT, prove, it is not as hard as you might think to lose that weight. But the rules for weight loss apply even more strongly if you are on HRT. Exercise! Don't aim too low! Don't expect fast loss!

you were 125 pounds in your early 20s, by 35 a weight of 129 pounds would be fine, by 45 a reasonable weight is 133 pounds, and by 55 about 137 pounds would be good going. Work this scale out now for yourself.

If you are within this target for your age, my advice is that you don't need to diet–use the Zest Plan on page 103 rather than the diet in Workshop 2. If you still feel you are fat, the shape assessment that follows will probably reveal that all you need is better muscle tone. However, if you have put on more than this "ideal gain," you probably would look better and younger shedding some weight.

Let's check you out further now, then, by working out your body mass index (BMI)–the modern equivalent of old-fashioned height/weight charts–to see just how overweight you might be.

ASSESSING YOUR WEIGHT AND SHAPE

The Body Mass Index

This involves using a calculator, so find yours and then here's what to do.

- **Start with your current weight in kilograms.**
  (To convert pounds into kilograms, divide by 2.2)

- **Convert your height into meters.**
  (To convert inches into meters, multiply by 0.025)

- **Square your height.**

- **Divide your weight by your squared height.**

THE ANSWER IS YOUR BMI.

Example:
You weigh 150 pounds.
(150 pounds ÷ 2.2 equals **68 kg**).

You are 5 feet 5 inches tall
(65 inches x 0.025 equals **1.62 meters**).

Your height squared
(1.62 x 1.62 is **2.62**).

Your BMI (**68** divided by **2.62** is **25.95**).
Round this up to 26.

The international classification for BMIs is:

Below 20	*Underweight*
20–25	*Acceptable weight range*
25–30	*Overweight*
30–40	*Obese (extremely overweight)*
Over 40	*Very obese (life-threatening obesity)*

Work out your own BMI here:

Current weight in kg ....

Height in meters ....

Height squared ....

Weight divided by height squared ....
Rounded up or down to the nearest half

MY BMI is...

Interpreting the Results

20 or below:
You should consider putting on some weight to bring your BMI up to between 20 and 25.

20–25:
If you are within the acceptable weight range and haven't put on more than the ideal gain explained on page 20 since your 20s, you don't need to diet. If you think you do, exercise is probably your answer. If your BMI is 20–25 and you *have* put on more than the ideal gain per decade, maybe you could do with losing a little, *but only if:*
- Your BMI is nearer 25 than 20 and
- Your WHR (explained right) is 0.80 or more.

25–30:
You probably need to lose weight–the nearer to 30 you are, the higher that likelihood is. If your BMI is over 25–but not much over–*here are some points to bear in mind*:
- If your weight is concentrated around your middle, but you have slim arms and legs, you likely need to diet.
- If you have heavy arms and legs, perhaps a large bust, but a reasonably slim midriff, you may not need to lose weight. I have seen two women of the same weight and height–one with a 33-inch waist, the other with a 28-inch waist. I advised the large-waisted woman to slim down, but not the other. The reason an "apple-shaped" woman should slim is because the apple shape is linked with heart disease more than the classic female "pear shape." And as women enter their menopause years they are more predisposed to develop an "apple shape," probably because of the hormonal changes that happen then.

If you are not sure if you are "apple shaped," an easy test is to divide your waist measurement by your hip measurement. If the resulting figure is over 0.80, you are an "apple."

This figure is your waist-to-hip ratio (WHR).

Over 30: You are definitely overweight and you need to slim. Start tomorrow. Workshop 2 will help you do that.

To Sum Up

- You want to be a healthy weight, not skinny.

- A healthy size can vary from person to person, but, in general, it is healthier to be shaped like a large pear than like an apple.

- If you are overweight, it is better to lose a sensible amount and keep it off, than to try to lose a lot and keep "yo-yoing."

Have years of yo-yo dieting ruined your metabolism?

It is a popular myth that if you spend years on and off diets, as many women now in their 30s, 40s, and 50s did, with weight going and then returning, your metabolism is affected so eventually you can no longer lose weight, no matter how much you reduce your food intake.

This, you will be pleased to hear, is not true. Researchers at the Dunn Nutrition Unit, the internationally respected obesity research center in Cambridge, England, have not found any evidence of metabolism being affected in this way in the scientific tests they conducted on yo-yo dieters.

What does happen is that as most people get older, they exercise less, their muscle mass diminishes, and, because muscle uses up more calories than other body tissue, the body's ability to burn calories and therefore shed weight (or stay slim) diminishes, too. If you've yo-yoed for years, you have been psychologically programmed to believe you will fail.

The rules for successfully losing weight–and keeping it off–as you get older are:

• Exercise.

• Do not aim for too low a weight.

• Accept a slow or steady weight-loss, rather than a rapid one.

• Eat a healthy diet while dieting–which is what you will find in the next workshop.

Your Shape

So, you are going to lose weight, if necessary, to get down to a size that is right for you now. But what about your body shape? By their late 30s and beyond, many women have lumps and bumps and saggy, baggy, or droopy bits on their bodies that aren't there just because of fat. They are due to lack of body tone and poor posture. You don't have to put up with them. *Take Off 10 Years in 10 Weeks* is here to help. But first take the shape test.

THE SHAPE TEST

Stand in front of a full-length mirror with no clothing on (make it a warm room!), with this book and a pen in hand, and complete the sections below:

1. Look at your body from top to toe and write down all the good things about it; all the things you like. Yes, you can find some. Everyone has good points. Don't be modest–no one else is going to see this. *Write them here, or if you prefer, in a notebook.*

2. Check out the things you can't alter. You have to be realistic. You can't alter: length of limbs, width of pelvis (hip bone structure), basic bone structure, shape of head, genetic tendency to a particular body shape, such as "pear." You can improve your basic shape, but not turn yourself into your genetic opposite. For example, if you are a "pear," with wide hips and big thighs and a small upper body and bust, you can reduce your hips and thighs somewhat and firm them up, and you can develop your upper body through exercise, but you can't get narrow hips and long skinny legs like a famous model.

Genetic Tendency to a Particular Body Type
There are three classifications of body type:
Ectomorph (long and skinny)
Endomorph (curvy and with a tendency to put on body fat easily)
Mesomorph (strong and muscular).

Most people have one of those three types dominant, with a little of one or even both of the others mixed in. *See if you can spot your dominant type.*

Ectomorphs find it hard to put on weight when young, but may gain weight when they get older; **endomorphs** are always having to watch what they eat to keep their weight down, and **mesomorphs** can stay slim and build muscle easily but need plenty of physical activity.
If your natural tendency is toward being an ectomorph, you are not be being realistic if your intention is to work out and build big muscles; be happy with a fit lean body. Be sensible.

Write down what your basic body type is here ➡

This is your body, accept those things you can't alter and learn to like–even love–the uniqueness of your body. In fact, go back and add to your list of things you like about your body, "I am unique!"

3. Look at the things you can change. If you are more than a little overweight, you may find it hard to differentiate between body fat and lack of body tone, but if you're not sure about any of the items below, check it.

Here is a list of body symptoms that can be altered through exercise, from top to toe. Go through the list and check any of them that apply to you:

Chin	❏ *double*
	❏ *saggy*
Neck	❏ *sunk into shoulders, seems too short*
Shoulders *front on*	❏ *very sloping, weak*
side on	❏ *rounded/hunched*
Upper arms	❏ *saggy, flabby underneath (lift them out to sides and shake)*
Bust	❏ *droopy*
Waist	❏ *thick*
Stomach *side on*	❏ *protruding*
Hips	❏ *flabby with love handles*
Bottom	❏ *flat*
	❏ *spread*
	❏ *droopy*
Thighs	❏ *spread*
Knees	❏ *fat*
Calves	❏ *lack definition*
Ankles	❏ *thick*
Feet	❏ *flat*

Don't be disheartened if you checked more than a few. It's almost as easy to shape up every bit of you as it is to shape up one bit! Workshops 3 and 4 and, to a lesser extent, Workshop 13 will transform you over the weeks ahead.

4. One last thing. Take a photo of yourself (put a swimsuit on if you like), front on and side on. You'll want to look back at it in 10 weeks' time and see just HOW much you've changed.

OUR PARTICIPANTS ASSESSED

Hilary has put on about 19 pounds since her 20s, has a BMI slightly over the ideal range of 20-25 with the surplus fat distributed quite evenly over her waist, hips, bottom, and thighs. I am going to set her target weight at about 133 pounds, which will bring her BMI down to just over 23. I would also like to see her lose an inch or two from around her waist; she wants to lose it from her buttocks, hips, thighs, and knees!

'"*I hate my knees – they are too fat to get into a pair of tapered pants I have!*"

Hilary swims regularly, but finds it hard going, and does not do any other exercise. The toning routine should firm her up all over and our stamina workshop (Workshop 14, page 105) will certainly increase her aerobic fitness.

HILARY, 43

Bust 35 inches
Waist 29½ inches
Hips 37½ inches
Thighs 23 inches
BMI 25.5
WHR .79
Weight 145 pounds
Height 5 feet 4 inches
General body tone "Soft and lacking in tone all over
Fitness level Slightly fit

Sue is just inside the top of the ideal BMI range and her WHR is fine, but she felt she wanted to lose a few pounds. "*I know my WHR seems OK, but the weight has mostly gone on around my tummy and, as I'm short-waisted, it looks even worse.*" We applied the "weight-gain-per-decade" criterion described earlier. In her mid 20s, Sue was 119 pounds. Now nearing 40, a reasonable normal weight gain would be 7 pounds, so the minimum she should aim to be is 126 pounds. However, I thought that might be unnecessarily low, so I set Sue's target at 128 pounds.

She will do plenty of abdominal exercises for her waist and stomach, as well as the Total Tone routine. She enjoys aerobic classes and will work out to a video our trainer, Louise, has prepared for all our participants, as well as fitting in tennis, walking, and an occasional session on a treadmill when she can.

SUE, 39

Bust 35½ inches
Waist 29½ inches
Hips 39½ inches
Thighs 22¼ inches
BMI 24.7
WHR .75
Weight 159 pounds
Height 5 feet 4 inches
General body tone Legs not too bad; abdomen, bottom, back, and arms quite poor
Fitness level Slightly fit

Pamela is slightly overweight according to the BMI, and her WHR is also poor–she's a classic "apple," with most of her surplus weight round her middle and with slim arms and legs. Add to that the fact that in her 20s she weighed 105 pounds, and has a tiny bone structure. We agreed Pamela should aim to lose about 15 pounds, bringing her BMI down to approximately 23, a good weight *if* she can reduce her waist and build a little muscle tone there and on her limbs.

Although Pam bowls every week and sometimes does a little gentle swimming and walking, none of this is enough to keep her toned or aerobically fit, or to maintain her bone density. We prescribed for her regular walking as detailed in the stamina workshop (Workshop 14, page 105), as well as Louise's aerobic tape. We have also given Pam a mini trampoline to work out on when she has spare time at home. This low-impact exercise is very good for older women.

PAMELA, 57

Bust 38½ inches
Waist 34½ inches
Hips 40 inches
Thighs 21½ inches
BMI 25.3
WHR .86
Weight 147 pounds
Height 5 feet 5 inches
General body tone Poor, especially abdomen, obliques, arms, and legs
Fitness level Very unfit

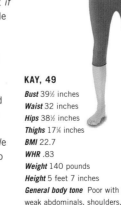

Kay, on paper, is an ideal weight, but she needs to redistribute this weight to look really good. She is a typical case of someone who is slim but has a low percentage of lean body tissue (muscle) and a high percentage of body fat. Her bust, waist, and abdomen carry most of this fat, and she may need to lose a few pounds to get her WHR down to below .80 and to get her top half more in proportion. Her limbs, particularly her legs, are slim but with little muscle definition, so she needs to work hard on her exercises to build up muscle in these areas. Her bust will also look firmer if she tones up her pectorals and shoulders.

Kay has never done any toning or aerobic exercise, so we need to build up her stamina. At 49 and smoking 20 cigarettes a day, Kay is worried this will be an impossible task–but we have assured her that if she eats sensibly, begins to exercise gently, and builds up to regular long sessions of walking, aerobics, and toning, as well as frequent sessions on her treadmill, she will achieve good results.

KAY, 49

Bust 39½ inches
Waist 32 inches
Hips 38½ inches
Thighs 17¼ inches
BMI 22.7
WHR .83
Weight 140 pounds
Height 5 feet 7 inches
General body tone Poor with weak abdominals, shoulders, arms, and legs
Fitness level Very unfit

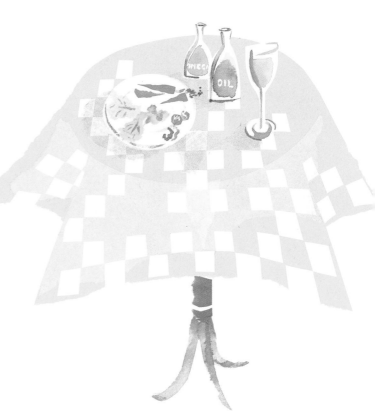

*S*o you need to lose some weight, and you have 10 weeks in which to do it. What can you expect to achieve? Following this plan, you can lose up to 20 pounds without fuss. Shedding that fat is pain free with the delicious meals and recipes in the Size-Wise Eating Plan (page 26). However, if you want to put on weight–or simply maintain your existing weight –turn to Workshop 13–Eating for Energy (page 100), where you'll find all the information you need on eating to shed the years instead.

WORKSHOP *2* YOUR PERSONAL EATING PLAN

*I*f your idea of a diet is deprivation and misery then think again. You can–indeed, you should–eat plenty while you lose those unwanted pounds of fat that have somehow accumulated over the years. What you need to do is start thinking of food as fuel: good fuel for your body. Give your body good-quality fuel and a minimum of junk, and it will respond by shedding weight without leaving you feeling tired, hungry, or depressed. A good diet–for weight loss or not–can help you to feel better and look better, too.

Good, nutritious food is one of the keys to youthful looks and vitality. The right diet can improve the condition and appearance of your skin, hair, eyes, and gums; and can help protect your health in many ways. You'll find more about healthy eating in Workshop 13 (page 100), but, for now, be assured the diet you'll find here is a healthy weight-loss diet, including all the nutrients your body needs for good health and well-being while you reshape your body.

The Size-Wise Eating Plan consists of a "flying-start" first week, followed by nine weeks of multichoice meals, allowing you to eat to suit your lifestyle and preferences. If you reach your target weight before the 10 weeks are up, simply move to the plan in Workshop 13. If you finish the 10 weeks and still have more to lose, just carry on.

Before you begin, remember losing weight is not just about choosing the right foods, but also about having the right attitude. So first read the eating tips that start in the next column.

Eating Tips and Information

1. The key to any successful weight-loss program is to get in touch with your appetite: this means learning to recognize real physical hunger and the other reasons why we eat–the wrong reasons! Beginning today, try these methods to drastically reduce the number of times in a day you eat for the wrong reasons:

Every time you are about to eat something, say, "Do I really need this? Am I truly hungry?" A lot of the time you will find yourself eating for other reasons–especially if the food, snack, or beverage in front of you is something fatty, sugary, or low in nutrients (a junk food). You may be bored or miserable, or maybe you're tempted to eat leftover food as you load the dishwasher. If you can resist food your body doesn't need for fuel, you're well on the way to winning. If you can't resist, don't feel guilty–after all, you have years of habits to unlearn, and every small victory, will eventually turn into a new habit for life.

When serving food, pay attention to your portion sizes. Examples of standard portion sizes are 3 or 4 ounces meat or poultry; 1 cup cooked pasta; 1 cup cooked leafy green vegetables, such as spinach; ½ cup starchy vegetables, such as corn or peas. We often pile much more on our plates than we really need. If you are still genuinely hungry when the plate is empty, you can always have more. If it is on the plate, however, the natural inclination is to eat it, even if you are quite satisfied. Not necessarily through gluttony—either we just don't think, or we've been told for years that leaving food is wasteful. It isn't necessary to measure out all your food, even on the Size-Wise plan. If you put slightly less on the plate than you think you'll want (with the exception of the "unlimited" foods we'll discuss later) and then eat *slowly*, you will often find you can cut portion sizes of calorie-rich foods by 25 percent.

As you get toward the end of your meal, learn to listen to your body. Have you had enough, even though there *is* some left? Learn to stop eating when you are satisfied. If you habitually have food left on the plate, you will know you should be serving yourself smaller portions.

Always remember the "good fuel" rule. When you *are* hungry, never feel guilty for eating "good fuel." This means fresh, natural foods such as salad greens, lightly cooked vegetables, fruits of all kinds, lean protein, low-fat dairy products, and natural carbohydrates such as whole-grain breads, rice, pasta, and beans. Good fuel is also, in moderation, fresh nuts and seeds, pure vegetable oils, and oily fish. (You'll learn more about good fuel in Workshop 13). Limit foods that are high in calories, sugar, and/or fat, but low on nutrients. Most cookies, cakes, pastries, and snack foods fall into this category. Bad fuel is also *too much* of certain foods that are okay if eaten occasionally. For example, cheddar cheese contains protein, calcium, and vitamins, but because it is high in saturated fat—and also in calories—a lot of it isn't good for your body or your diet. The Size-Wise plan gives you a diet that is very high in good fuel and low on bad fuel.

2. Eat regularly—from when you wake up to when you have your evening meal. Don't allow more than three hours to go by without eating something. Yes, this *is* a diet . . . but our bodies appreciate and respond to regular meals. I am not talking about five big meals a day—nor even five small meals—but breakfast, lunch, an evening meal, and two small snacks in between. These will keep you from feeling hungry and therefore keep you happy—which is what will make you stick to the plan. So don't skip meals: eat everything you are allowed. If you are one of the many people who has spent the past 20 years doing all the wrong things to diet, you may find my program strange at first and feel you won't lose weight while eating so much. But you will!

40-PLUS SLIMMING THE FACTS

Many people complain to me that they find it much harder to lose weight since they have been in their 40s or 50s. This can be true–but it doesn't have to be. The reasons we tend to put on weight as we get older, and also find it harder to shift the pounds, are twofold. Over the age of 35, our muscles (lean body tissue) very gradually begin to lose their mass. In other words, we begin to lose lean tissue, and the loss gradually speeds up over the years. As lean tissue is much more metabolically active than other body tissue, this means that gradually our metabolic rate (the rate at which we burn up calories) slows down. It is estimated that, all other things being equal, we need to eat 50 fewer calories a day for every five years over the age of 30 if we are, to maintain our weight. At 50 you need 200 calories a day less than you did at 30! It follows that at 50 you would also need to reduce the calories in a weight-loss diet by 200 a day to lose weight as quickly as someone 20 years younger. Added to that is the fact that as we get older, almost all of us exercise less. Exercise burns calories and speeds up the metabolism. So less exercise is one more reason why older people need fewer calories. Due to hormonal changes, women may also put on several pounds during menopause, or while on hormone replacement therapy, even without changing their eating habits. But don't be depressed. Though the surplus pounds are there, they are *not* there permanently, as you are about to discover. There are two solutions: the older you are, you must learn to be happier with a gradual weight loss. After all, even half a pound a week equals nearly 26 pounds in a year. And, whatever your age, you *must* exercise regularly. This helps to keep lean tissue density *and* burns calories. It's also vital not to work toward too low a body weight–something you will realize after your weight assessment in Workshop 1.

On the Size-Wise Eating Plan, women of 50-plus may be able to lose 10 pounds or more in the 10 weeks; women of 40-plus 12 pounds or more, and women of 30-plus 15 pounds or more.

Instructions applicable for all 10 weeks

**Plan what you are going to eat at least a day in advance;
shop up to a week in advance if possible.**

DAILY MILK ALLOWANCE

Every day on the plan you have an allowance of up to 2 cups (500 ml) of skim milk.
If you don't want this, have 1½ cups (250 ml) plain yogurt instead. Dairy products are important
sources of calcium, important in preventing osteoporosis, as are broccoli, kale, canned sardines,
and fortified citrus juices and punches.

UNLIMITEDS

*Every day on the diet you can eat or drink any of the following
in addition to the meals, snacks and extras.*

Foods

- all fresh vegetables *except starchy vegetables such as potatoes and sweet potatoes, which should only be eaten as stated within the plan*
- all fresh salad ingredients. In fact, you should eat as much fresh salad and lightly cooked or raw vegetables as possible, both at lunch time and in the evening. Bake, steam, lightly boil, braise, or microwave to avoid adding fat during cooking. Salads can be dressed with any of the unlimited condiments above. Balsamic vinegar is excellent as it is sweet and flavorful, or use a teaspoon of reduced-fat mayonnaise mixed with a little low-fat plain yogurt.

Drinks

- water
- mineral water
- weak black tea or coffee (or with milk from allowance)
- unsweetened fruit and herbal teas
- unsweetened fruit and vegetable juices.
- Avoid diet sodas and soft drinks as they have little or no nutritional benefit.

Condiments

- all fresh or dried herbs and spices
- salt (use sparingly)
- pepper
- lemon juice; lime juice
- chili sauce
- mustard
- Worcestershire sauce
- reduced-sodium soy sauce
- vinegar
- sour pickles such as gherkins and onions
- fat-free dressing
- tomato paste

EATING PROFILE

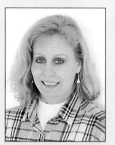

Virtually vegetarian, **Hilary** has been eating plenty of fruit and vegetables, pasta, rice, and other carbohydrates, but I found her diet low in protein, iron, and particularly calcium because she eats few dairy products. Her one main "vice" is chocolate. "The lack of calcium in my diet does worry me," she said, "because I don't want to risk osteoporosis as I get older."

I have given Hilary a daily chocolate allowance and explained the best sources of calcium.

By the end of Week 2, she had already lost 4 pounds and was already noticing that she had more energy.

FRUIT CHOICE

When "fruit choice" is mentioned within the plans, choose one medium piece
(one apple) or two small pieces (two plums) or one average portion (a medium plate
of strawberries) of your choice. Bananas should be limited to one per day maximum and
should be small. Eat as much citrus fruit as you can (within reason, very high quantities
of citrus and some other fruits can cause digestive problems). Be adventurous!
Apples and bananas are marvelous foods, but there is so much more out
there waiting for you to try–exotic fruits such as mango,
papaya, and starfruit.

*Always remember:
fresh vegetables and salads
are unlimited
– eat as much of them as you want!*

THE SIZE-WISE FLYNG START—WEEK 1 ONLY

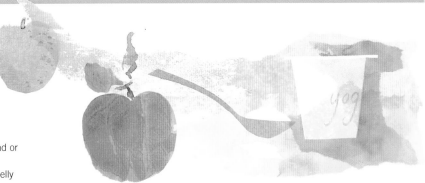

BREAKFAST

- Pick a Fruit Choice. Cut, segment, or stir your fruit into ¹/₂ cup (125 ml) low-fat plain yogurt or low-fat cottage cheese.
- Add a handful of high fiber cereal
- Serve with ¹/₂ cup (125 ml) orange juice.

MID-MORNING

- Choose one of the following:
  - 1 whole wheat crisp roll, plain or with fruit spread or sugar-free jelly
  - 1 rye crispbread with fruit spread or sugar-free jelly
  - 5 dried apricots, peaches, or prunes
  - 1 apple
  - crudités dipped in a little reduced-fat mayonnaise mixed with low-fat plain yogurt

LUNCH

either

Sandwich Lunch

- Using 2 slices whole-grain bread and a little reduced-fat mayonnaise, butter, or margarine, make a sandwich with one of the following fillings:
  - 3½ ounces (100 g) tuna canned in water
  - 1 hard-cooked egg
  - 2 ounces (50 g) reduced-fat cheese
  - 2 ounces (50 g) lean roast chicken
  - 1½ ounces (40 g) Brie or Edam cheese
  - plus unlimited salad
  - *1 Fruit Choice and 1 low-fat, plain or artifically sweetened yogurt*

or

Salad Lunch

- Make a large salad and have it with one of the sandwich fillings above, plus 1 whole-wheat roll or 2 slices whole-grain bread followed by 1 Fruit Choice and 1 yogurt as above.

or

Hot Lunch

- Have a large baked potato filled with one of the following:
  - ⅓ cup (6 tablespoons) baked beans
  - ¼ cup (50 g) low-fat cream cheese (melt in microwave if desired)
  - 2 ounces (50 g) tuna canned in water, drained and mixed with ¹/₃ cup (50 g) beans and 1 teaspoon reduced-fat mayonnaise
- OR have 2 slices bread as above, toasted and topped with one of the following:
  - ⅓ cup (6 tablespoons) baked beans
  - 1 poached egg
- plus 1 Fruit Choice and 1 low-fat plain or artificially sweetened diet yogurt.

MID-AFTERNOON

- Fruit Choice

EVENING

- Choose one of these, plainly cooked; common dietary guidelines define a portion of meat or poultry as 3 to 4 ounces (75-100 g):
  - turkey cutlet
  - chicken portion (skin removed)
  - white fish portion
  - small trout or salmon steak
  - 2 slices lean roast meat
  - 1 vegetable burger
  - omelet of 2 large eggs
- Add unlimited salad and/or vegetables, plus medium (¾ to 1 cup/200 g)) portion plainly cooked pasta, potato, rice, or other grain, or 2 ounces (50 g) bread.
- Add any of the following:
  - 1-2 tablespoons fat-free sauce or gravy
  - 1 level teaspoon reduced-fat mayonnaise or pickle relish

NOTE: *For a change, thinly slice your protein, vegetables, and salad and use your unlimited condiments plus 1 level teaspoon honey to make a stir-fry, preparing the wok or pan with a light coating of nonstick vegetable oil cooking spray, and adding a ¼ to ½ cup defatted broth to make a sauce.*

Size-Wise Tips

Entertaining?

This is easier than eating out, as you are in control of what you prepare and serve. Choose from the recipes at the end of this workshop or scour books, weight-loss magazines, and libraries for lowfat, low-cal recipes. Don't be afraid to try new ideas—apart from your makeup, hair, and clothes, nothing dates you more than an outdated repertoire of recipes! As long as you don't want to entertain every other evening, you can still lose weight by following the plan extra diligently for the rest of the time.

Vegetarian?

That's fine—there are plenty of vegetarian choices within the meal selections. There are also several vegetarian recipes, and others that can easily be adapted.

THE SIZE-WISE EATING PLAN—WEEKS 2 TO 10

EXTRAS

EVERY DAY you may choose one or two of the following in addition to the rest of your diet, as explained in the instructions:

- 1 glass dry/medium-dry wine

- 1 tablespoon butter or oil

- ½ cup (125 ml) low-fat ice cream

- 1 tablespoon fat-free salad dressing

- 2 tablespoons low-fat sour cream

- ⅓ cup (6 tablespoons) reduced-calorie pudding

- 1 English muffin

Size-Wise Tips

Eating out?

No one expects you to live like a hermit while you lose weight. When eating out, you can control the number of calories you eat by choosing a main course and either an appetizer or a dessert by having fresh fruit for both appetizer and dessert; by declining bread and butter; by avoiding main courses that are obviously high in fat, such as pastry-wrapped dishes and anything fried.

NOTE: Milk allowance, Unlimiteds, and Fruit Choices as Week 1.
INSTRUCTIONS: Every day you will be eating a Breakfast, a Mid-morning Snack, a Lunch, a Mid-afternoon Snack, and an Evening Meal, plus one or two items from a choice of Extras. **If you have 15 pounds (7.5 kg) or less to lose:** Choose a *small break-fast* and pick just *one* Extra a day from the list. **If you have more than 15 pounds (7.5 kg) to lose:** Choose a *large breakfast* and pick *two* Extras a day from the list. Now all you have to do is select your meals from the lists each day–and see the pounds melt away!

COLD BREAKFAST

Small

- Same breakfast as Week 1.
- 1½ ounces (40 g) muesli with milk from allowance; 1 Fruit Choice.
- 1 ounce (25 g) unsweetened high fiber cereal of choice with milk from allowance; 1 large banana or 2 Fruit Choices.
- 1 ounce (25 g) unsweetened high fiber cereal of choice with milk from allowance and ½ cup (3½ oz) diced fruit of choice mixed in, plus 5 chopped dried apricots or prunes.
- ½ cup (125 ml) low-fat plain yogurt with 1 teaspoon honey and 1 Fruit Choice.
- 1½ slices bread, preferably whole grain, with a little reduced-calorie butter or margarine and 2 teaspoons low-sugar jam or marmalade; 1 artificially sweetened fruit yogurt; 1 Fruit Choice.
- 1 ounce (25 g) unsweetened high fiber cereal of choice with milk from allowance, 1 small slice bread with a little reduced-fat butter or margarine and I teaspoon low-sugar jam, marmalade, or fruit spread; ½ grapefruit or 1 kiwi fruit.

Large

- 1½ ounces (40 g) unsweetened high fiber cereal of choice with skim milk to cover and 1 Fruit Choice (chopped in if desired); 1 slice bread (preferably wholegrain) with a little reduced-calorie butter or margarine and 1 tea-spoon low-sugar jam, marmalade, or fruit spread.
- 2 ounces (50 g) no-added-sugar muesli with skim milk to cover; 1 Fruit Choice.
- 2 slices whole-grain bread with a little reduced-calorie butter or margarine and 4 tea-spoons low-sugar preserves; 1 large banana *or* 1 Fruit Choice, plus 1 plain or low-fat artificially sweetened yogurt.
- Unlimited fresh fruit of choice or up to 2 ounces (50 g) chopped mixed dried fruit, mixed into ½ cup (125 ml) plain yogurt with 1 level teaspoon brown sugar or honey, 1 ounce unsweetened high fiber cereal of choice or ½ ounce (15 g) muesli.

HOT BREAKFAST

Small

- 1 slice toast with a little reduced-calorie butter or margarine, topped with 1 small banana, sliced or mashed with a little lemon juice and cinnamon; 1 artificially sweetened low-fat fruit yogurt.
- 1 slice toast, spread with a little low-fat cream cheese and topped with 2 or 3 halved tomatoes, broiled, sautéed using vegetable oil cooking spray, or baked; 1 Fruit Choice.
- 1 medium egg, boiled or poached, with 1 slice toast and a little reduced-calorie butter or mar-garine; 1 Fruit Choice.
- 1 average bowl of oatmeal made with equal parts water and skim milk; 1 teaspoon brown sugar; 1 Fruit Choice.
- 1 slice toast with a little reduced-calorie butter or margarine, topped with ¼ cup (4 table-spoons) baked beans; 1 citrus fruit.

Large

- 1 egg, poached or fried in a pan prepared with vegetable oil cooking spray; ¼ cup (4 table-spoons) baked beans; 1 slice lean turkey bacon, broiled or fried until crisp; 1 broiled tomato; 1 small slice wholegrain bread with a little reduced-fat butter or margarine; ½ grapefruit.
- ¾ cup (200 g) baked beans on 1 slice toast; 1 Fruit Choice.
- ½ cup oatmeal made with equal parts water and skim milk with 1 teaspoon sugar or honey; 1 slice bread with a little reduced-calorie butter or margarine; 1 Fruit Choice.
- Fruit compote and yogurt: simmer cups mixed dried fruit in water to cover until the fruit is ten-der and a rich fruity juice develops. Serve 5 to 6 pieces of the fruit and some of the juice with ½ cup (125 ml) low-fat plain yogurt, a handful of whole-grain cereal flakes, and 1 teaspoon honey; ⅔ cup (200 ml) unsweetened orange juice.

PACKED LUNCHES

- 2 slices whole-grain bread with a little reduced-fat butter or margarine filled with plenty of fresh salad and one of the following:
  - 1 hard-cooked egg and 1 teaspoon reduced-fat mayonnaise
  - 3 ounces shelled cooked shrimp and 1 teaspoon reduced-fat mayonnaise
  - 2 slices lean ham and 1 teaspoon prepared mustard or pickle relish
  - 2 ounces (50 g) lean cooked chicken or turkey and 1 teaspoon reduced-fat mayonnaise
  - 1 ounce (25 g) Edam, Brie, Gouda, Jarlsberg, or Blue cheese
  - 1½ ounces (40 g) reduced-fat Cheddar or other cheese
  - 2 ounces (50 g) smoked salmon, lemon juice, and black pepper
  - 1 ounce (25 g) prosciutto ham and 4 or 5 cooked asparagus spears

Plus (with any of above selections)
1 Fruit Choice and either 1 pack low-calorie dried soup or 1 artificially sweetened diet yogurt, or low-fat cottage cheese

- 1 large whole-grain roll with a little reduced-fat butter or margarine, filled with plenty of fresh salad and one of the following:
  - 1 ounce (25 g) cheddar and 1 teaspoon pickle relish.
  - 1 thin slice extra-lean ham and 1 tablespoon low-fat cottage cheese
  - 3 ounces (75 g) lean cooked chicken (skin removed)
  - 2 ounces (50 g) lean roast beef and 1 teaspoon horseradish
  - 2 ounces (50 g) fresh poached salmon or canned salmon and 1 teaspoon reduced-fat mayonnaise
- 1 portion Smoked Trout Pâté (page 31)
Plus 1 large banana with any of the above.
- 1 pita bread filled with plenty of fresh mixed salad and one of the following:
  - 2 tablespoons hummus
  - 1 tablespoon taramasalata
  - 2 ounces (50 g) Feta cheese, crumbled
  - 3½ ounces (100 g) tuna canned in water and 2 or 3 chopped pitted black olives

Plus 2 Fruit Choices with any of the above.

- 1 cup Lentil and Vegetable Soup (page 32), 1 whole-grain roll; 1 low-fat or artificially sweetened yogurt; 1 Fruit Choice
- 1 deli sandwich totaling 300 calories or less and containing plenty of lettuce and tomato (restrict to occasional use).
- 1 portion homemade Mixed Bean and Pasta Salad (page 33); 1 large banana.

COLD LUNCHES
AND SNACKS

- Any of the packed lunch ideas–have more lettuce and tomato on your plate than you would get in a sandwich.
- 1 portion of Fresh Tuna Salad (page 33) served with 1 small whole-grain roll with a little reduced-fat mayonnaise, butter, or margarine.
- Salad made by combining 2 ounces (50 g) crumbled Feta cheese with 1 large chopped tomato, chopped cucumber, crisp lettuce, 2 green onions, 2 black olives, and a little diced red bell pepper in fat-free salad dressing to taste; 1 mini pita; 2 Fruit Choices or 1 banana.
- Low-fat Submarine: 3-inch (7.5-cm) slice whole-wheat French bread with a little reduced-calorie butter or margarine; 1½ ounces (40 g) reduced-fat Cheddar cheese *or* other reduced-fat hard cheese; large mixed salad with fat-free oil-and-vinegar dressing or a dash of balsamic vinegar; celery sticks, 2 teaspoons sweet pickle relish; pickled onions.
NOTE: *You can have 2 slices extra-lean ham or corned beef or 3½ ounces (100 g) tuna canned in water or 3 ounces (75 g) shelled shrimp instead of the cheese.*
- Low-fat coleslaw with 1 slice bread and a little reduced-fat butter or margarine, plus either 2 ounces (50 g) lean cooked chicken or low-fat cheese, lean ham, or vegetarian pâté.
- A chicken and fruit salad made by combining: ½ cup (3 oz) diced cooked chicken with 2 ounces (50 g) each diced melon, orange, and apple, tossed in 2 tablespoons reduced-fat mayonnaise mixed with 1 tablespoon skim milk and ½ teaspoon mild curry powder; 1 small whole-grain roll with reduced-fat butter or margarine; 1 artificially sweetened low-fat yogurt.
- 1 portion Gazpacho Soup (page 32); 2 slices whole-grain bread; 1 ounce (25 g) Brie or Edam.
- 1 portion Red Pepper Dip (page 31) with plenty of raw veggies, 2 ounces (50 g) French bread; 1 banana; 1 Fruit Choice.
NOTE: *You can substitute 3 dark rye crisps, or rye crisp toast for any one slice of bread in the lunches.*

HOT LUNCHES
AND SNACKS

- The Gazpacho Soup (page 32) meal from packed lunches.
- ¾ cup (200 g) baked beans on 1 large slice whole-grain toast; 1 banana *or* 2 scoops low-fat ice cream; 1 kiwi fruit or small portion of fresh berries.
- 1¼ cups (300 ml) fresh vegetable, carrot, or lentil soup; 1 whole-grain roll; 1 small English muffin with a little reduced-calorie butter or margarine or ½ cup (125 ml) fruit yogurt; 1 banana or 2 Fruit Choices.
- 1 large baked potato filled with ¼ cup (4 tablespoons) baked beans; *or* Chili Chicken (*page 34*); lots of lettuce and tomato; 1 level tablespoon grated Parmesan cheese.
- 1 large baked potato filled with 2 tablespoons creamy dressing made by mixing together equal quantities of reduced-fat mayonnaise and low-fat plain yogurt topped with 1 teaspoon grated Parmesan cheese. Serve with plenty of salad.
- 1 small individual pizza crust spread with 1 tablespoon pizza sauce, covered with 4 thin slices of low-fat mozzarella cheese *or* 2 tablespoons low-fat shredded mozzarella and finished with slices of tomato, mushroom, and pepper; bake until bubbling and golden. Serve with plenty of lettuce and tomatoes.
- 1 frozen cheese-and-tomato French bread pizza; a lot of salad; 1 Fruit Choice.
- 2 medium eggs, scrambled with a little skim milk and seasoning in a nonstick skillet or use vegetable oil cooking spray on 2 slices of whole-grain bread with a little reduced-fat butter or margarine; 1 banana or 1 citrus fruit and 1 other Fruit Choice.

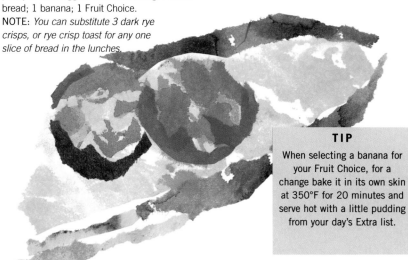

TIP
When selecting a banana for your Fruit Choice, for a change bake it in its own skin at 350°F for 20 minutes and serve hot with a little pudding from your day's Extra list.

MAIN MEALS

Red Meat and Poultry

- 1 medium lean pork cutlet, broiled; 8 ounces (225 g) new potatoes with 1 teaspoon butter; a lot of vegetables; some apple sauce if liked.
- 4 ounces (110 g) boneless pork or lamb, cubed and threaded on a skewer with cubes of red bell pepper and chunks of red onion, brushed with oil and broiled; serve with 5 tablespoons boiled rice, 2 tablespoons heated Italian bottled tomato sauce, and lots of salad. *TIP: If you have time, marinate the meat first for a while in a little soy sauce or red wine.*

- Average-sized chicken portion, skin removed, and coated in a mixture of low-fat plain yogurt and mild curry, tikka, or tandoori powder (not paste), broiled or baked; serve with ⅓ cup (5 tablespoons) boiled rice, 1 teaspoon chutney, and a green salad.
- Average-sized chicken portion, skin removed broiled, and served with 7 ounces (200 g) new potatoes, plenty of "free" vegetables, and low-fat gravy or 2 tablespoons Pesto Tomato Sauce (page 35); 1 Fruit Choice.
- 1 small chicken breast portion, skin removed, sliced, and stir-fried with a selection of vegetables in 1 tablespoon corn oil; add seasonings of choice, such as soy sauce, ginger, chili, five-spice powder; 1 cup (200 g) cooked noodles, rice, or pasta.
- Any frozen meal labeled "low-fat" and containing 400 calories or less; large mixed salad *or* 2 or 3 vegetables; 1 Fruit Choice.
- 4 ounces (110 g) lean roast beef or 5 ounces (140 g) lean roast chicken; serve with small baked potato, several unlimited vegetables, and 2 tablespoons wine gravy or skimmed pan juices and 1 teaspoon condiment of choice. *TIP: Toss a selection of root vegetables in 1 teaspoon olive oil and roast for 45 minutes at 375°F, turning once. Count the oil as your day's Extra.*

- 1 portion Chili Chicken (page 34) serve with ½ cup (6 tablespoons) steamed basmati or other fragrant rice; large salad.
- 1 portion Chicken, Lime, and Mango Brochettes (page 35); serve with ½ cup (6 tablespoons) steamed long-grain brown and wild rices; green salad.

Fish

- 6 ounces (175 g) white fish fillet, cooked without added fat; served with 6 ounces (175 g) potatoes, boiled, mashed with skim milk, or baked potato, plus 6 ounces (175 g) peas, broccoli, carrots, or other suitable vegetables, and 1 teaspoon sauce of choice.
- 1 small trout sautéed in nonstick vegetable oil cooking spray and served with 1 teaspoon flaked toasted almonds and lemon juice; potatoes, and vegetables.
- Monkfish or swordfish kabob: cube 7 ounces (200 g) monkfish fillet and thread on kabob skewer with tomato, 1 slice lean bacon cut into cubes, onion slices, and zucchini cubes. Brush with a little oil and broil. Serve with 2-3 tablespoons tomato sauce and ⅓ cup (4 tablespoons) plain boiled rice or noodles, and lots of salad.
- 5 ounces (150 g) salmon steak, topped with 1 tablespoon prepared fresh pesto sauce and broiled on a baking sheet for 7-8 minutes; 7 ounces (200 g) new potatoes; peas or broccoli.
- 1 portion Spiced Salmon Fishcakes (*page 34*); large mixed salad; 1 Fruit Choice.
- 1 portion Whole Fish, Catalan Style (*page 34*), 5 ounces (150 g) new potatoes; large mixed salad.
- Salmon and Broccoli Risotto: Allow ¼ cup (50 g) dried weight arborio rice per person; toss rice in nonstick skillet with 1 tablespoon (15 g) butter to coat; add ⅔ cup (140 ml) well-flavored vegetable, chicken or fish broth per person; simmer, stirring and adding more broth as needed. When rice is almost tender, stir in ½ cup (75 g) parboiled broccoli florets and 3 ounces (75 g) flaked cooked fresh or canned salmon per person. Stir and serve with chopped parsley when rice is tender and still moist, seasoning to taste.

Pasta, Eggs, and Vegetables

- 2 ounces (50 g) dried pasta of your choice, boiled and topped with either ⅓ cup (5 tablespoons) bottled or home made tomato sauce (page 35) and 1 tablespoon grated Parmesan cheese. Add sliced button mushrooms if you like, or top with 2 tablespoons prepared pesto sauce, mixed with 1 large finely chopped fresh tomato and 1 small handful of pine nuts (optional) *or* ½ cup (100 g) any pasta sauce that doesn't contain cream. Serve with a lot of salad.
- 2-egg omelet cooked in nonstick pan prepared with vegetable oil cooking spray, and filled with either sliced button mushrooms or a few shrimp; serve with a 3-inch (7.5-cm) slice French bread and salad.
- 2 ounces (50 g) dried weight medium egg-thread noodles cooked according to package instructions and tossed with a selection of thinly sliced vegetables stir-fried in 1 tablespoon corn oil, soy sauce, and 1 tablespoon bottled black or yellow bean sauce. Add a little stock for a moister stir-fry. Add 2 ounces (50 g) lean cooked chicken, turkey, or tofu, and stir-fry for 1 to 2 minutes longer before serving.
- Any pasta, rice, or vegetarian frozen meal labeled "low-fat" and containing 400 calories or less; large mixed salad or vegetables; 1 Fruit Choice.

**Limit
convenience meals
to one a week
maximum.**

- Cheese and tomato pizza for one; large mixed salad.
- One 4-ounce (110 g) vegetable burger; 1 whole-grain roll *or* 7 ounces (200 g) new potatoes; vegetables of choice or large salad; 1 teaspoon relish of choice; 1 banana.
- 1 portion Cantonese Vegetable Stir-Fry (page 33); ¾ cup (50 g) steamed brown rice; 1 banana.
- 1 portion Goulash of Winter Vegetables and Beans (page 33); ⅔ cup (40 g) steamed brown rice.
- 1 portion Pasta with Pesto Tomato Sauce (page 35); green salad.
- 1 portion Pasta Primavera (page 35).

RECIPES

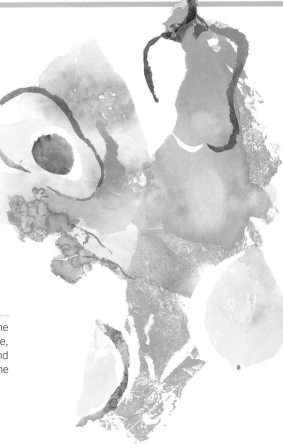

All recipes serve four, but most quantities can be halved to serve two. If cooking for one, some dishes can be frozen, so you can cook for two or four and freeze the surplus. Dishes suitable for freezing are marked with an asterisk (❄).

AVOCADO LIME DIP

125 calories; 12g fat per serving;
good source of vitamin E

....

- •*2 ripe medium avocados*
- •*juice of 1 large lime*
- •*few drops hot-pepper sauce*
- •*pinch* each *salt and black pepper*
- •*chopped fresh cilantro leaves, to garnish (optional)*

....

Peel and pit the avocados and mash the flesh in a small bowl. Add the lime juice, hot-pepper sauce, salt, and pepper and combine well. Serve garnished with the cilantro leaves, if you like.

The dip can also be used as a crisp-bread or open-faced sandwich topping, and will keep in an airtight container in the refrigerator for a few days if covered completely with a thin film of olive oil. Skim the oil off before serving.

SMOKED TROUT PÂTÉ ❄

130 calories; 9g fat per serving

good source of
omega-3 oils, protein,
calcium, vitamin B₃

....

- •*6 ounces (175 g) smoked trout fillet*
- •*½ cup (100 g) reduced-fat cottage cheese*
- •*2 tablespoons plain low-fat yogurt*
- •*juice of ½ lemon*
- •*2 teaspoons horseradish sauce*
- •*pinch* each *salt and black pepper*
- •*chopped fresh parsley or dill, to garnish*

....

Put all the ingredients except the garnish in a food processor or blender and blend until smooth.

Adjust the seasoning, chill, and serve garnished with the parsley or dill.

RED PEPPER DIP

65 calories; 2g fat per serving

good source of
beta-carotene, vitamin C, fiber

....

- •*2 large red bell peppers, halved and seeded*
- •*½ cup (100 g) low-fat mayonnaise*
- •*few drops hot-pepper sauce*
- •*pinch* each *salt and black pepper*
- •*paprika, to garnish*

....

Place the peppers on a baking sheet, skin side up. Broil for about 10 minutes, without turning, until the skins have charred. Remove from heat and place in a brown paper bag. Leave for 5 minutes; the skins will come off easily (leave a few black bits of skin on the peppers to add a pleasant smoky flavor to the dip). Chop the peppers coarsely and place in a food processor or blender with remaining ingredients except the paprika. Blend to a smooth consistency. Chill and serve sprinkled with paprika.

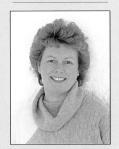

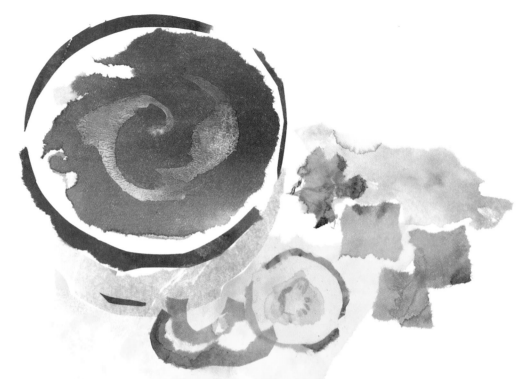

LENTIL AND VEGETABLE SOUP *

200 calories; 5g fat per serving

good source of
fiber, magnesium, iron, vitamin E,
B-group vitamins, vitamin C

- 1 tablespoon sunflower or canola oil
- 1 large onion, finely chopped
- 1–2 teaspoons curry powder (optional)
- 5 cups (1 liter) defatted vegetable or chicken broth
- generous ½ cup (110 g) uncooked brown or green lentils
- 1 large leek, cleaned and chopped
- 1 large parsnip, peeled and chopped
- 2 medium carrots, chopped
- ⅔ cup (100 g) peeled and chopped rutabaga or sweet potato
- ⅔ cup (100 g) peeled, seeded, and chopped butternut squash
- 1 large potato, peeled and chopped
- 2 celery stalks, chopped
- 2 teaspoons tomato paste
- 1 teaspoon sun-dried tomato paste (optional)
- pinch each salt and black pepper

Heat the oil in a large saucepan and sauté the onion until soft. Add the curry powder, if using, and stir for a minute or two. Add the broth and lentils and bring to a boil; reduce the heat and simmer for 45 minutes or until lentils are tender.

Add the remaining ingredients and simmer for another 45 minutes or until all the vegetables are tender.

Transfer half the soup to a food processor or blender and blend until smooth. Return the blended soup to the pan, heat through, and serve.

WATERCRESS AND PEA SOUP *

112 calories; 4g fat per serving

good source of
vitamin C, beta-carotene, fiber, iron

- 1 tablespoon (15 g) butter
- 1 medium sweet red or white onion or 4–5 shallots, peeled and chopped
- 3¾ cups (825 ml) defatted vegetable or chicken broth
- 2¼ cups (325 g) shelled fresh peas or frozen baby peas
- 2 bunches watercress, picked over and large stems removed
- pinch each of salt and black pepper
- 1 tablespoon chopped fresh mint

Melt the butter in a large saucepan and sauté the onion or shallots until soft. Add the broth, peas, and watercress and bring to a boil; reduce heat and simmer for 10 to 15 minutes.

Season to taste with salt and pepper, then put the soup in a food processor or blender and blend until almost smooth (only a few seconds). Return to the pan and reheat, stirring the mint in for the last minute.

Variations: You can cook the same recipe using fresh parsley instead of watercress. You can also add some boiled russet baking potato to this or the lentil soup recipe for thicker, more substantial soups. Two medium potato chunks will add about 25 calories and no fat per portion.

GAZPACHO SOUP

120 calories; 4g fat per serving

good source of
beta-carotene, vitamin C, fiber

- 1 large green bell pepper, seeded and finely diced
- 1 pound (450 g) cucumbers, peeled and finely diced
- 1 small mild Spanish onion, peeled and finely diced
- 1 garlic clove, minced
- 1 can (16 ounces/450 g) peeled plum tomatoes or 6 ripe tomatoes, peeled, seeded, and chopped, including juice
- 1 tablespoon red wine vinegar
- 1 tablespoon olive oil
- 3 tablespoons tomato paste
- pinch chili powder or dash hot-pepper sauce
- 2 tablespoons chopped fresh parsley
- 2 slices whole-wheat bread

Reserve 1 tablespoon each of the bell pepper, cucumber, and onion. In a food processor or blender, in batches, if necessary, process the remaining ingredients except the parsley and bread for garnish. Add water, as desired, to make a fairly thick soup. Stir well and chill for an hour or two in the refrigerator.

Make croutons by cutting the bread into ½-inch cubes. Put on a baking sheet and bake at 375°F (190°C), tossing a few times, until golden and crisp.

Ladle the chilled soup into bowls, garnish each with a little of the reserved bell pepper, cucumber, and onion, and a sprinkling of parsley and croutons.

BEAN AND PASTA SALAD

265 calories; 5g fat per serving

good source of
fiber, protein, vitamin C

- 1½ cups (150 g) uncooked small pasta shells, boiled and drained
- 1 can (19 ounces/525 g) black beans, rinsed and drained
- 1 ripe medium tomato, seeded and chopped
- 4 green onions, chopped
- 2 tablespoons chopped fresh parsley
- 5 tablespoons fat-free vinaigrette dressing
- 1 tablespoon olive oil
- pinch sugar

Toss together the pasta shells, black beans, tomato, green onions, and parsley in a salad bowl. In a small bowl, combine the dressing, olive oil, and sugar. Pour dressing over the salad, stir gently, and serve.

NUTTY RICE SALAD

350 calories; 8g fat per serving

good source of
B vitamins, vitamin E, fiber, protein

- 1 cup (200 g) uncooked brown rice, steamed and cooled slightly
- 4 rings fresh pineapple (or canned in juice), chopped
- 1 red apple, cored and chopped (including skin)
- 1 tablespoon pine nuts
- 2 tablespoons toasted slivered almonds
- 1 large banana, peeled and sliced
- 7 ounces (220 g) cooked chicken, skin removed and diced, or 7 ounces (200 g) firm tofu, cut into chunks
- ½ cup (8 tablespoons) fat-free vinaigrette dressing
- 1 tablespoon chopped fresh cilantro leaves, to garnish (optional)

Combine all the ingredients except the cilantro. Serve immediately, garnished with the cilantro.

FRESH TUNA SALAD

260 calories; 6.5g fat per serving

good source of
fiber, vitamin E, omega-3 oils, vitamin C, B-group vitamins, calcium, protein, iron

- olive oil cooking spray
- 14 ounces (400 g) fresh tuna steak, cut into chunks
- 4 Bibb lettuce heads or 2 Boston lettuces
- 1 can (15 ounces/425 g) cannellini beans, rinsed and drained
- 1 yellow bell pepper, seeded and sliced
- 8 black pitted olives, halved
- 1 small red onion, thinly sliced
- 12 cherry tomatoes
- 2 hard-cooked eggs, shelled and quartered
- ¼ cup (4 tablespoons) fat-free vinaigrette dressing

Spray a large nonstick skillet with the oil spray and heat. When hot, add tuna chunks and sear outsides until golden. Reduce heat and continue cooking for a minute or two until the fish is just tender. Let cool slightly.

Meanwhile, quarter the lettuces, removing any discolored outer leaves. Arrange on a serving platter. Add the beans, tuna, bell pepper, olives, onion, cherry tomatoes, and eggs in separate piles on the platter between the lettuce quarters.

Spoon the dressing over and serve.

NOTE: *Good-quality canned tuna can be used. There is no need to fry it.*

CANTONESE VEGETABLE STIR-FRY

126 calories; 6g fat per serving

good source of
fiber, protein, vitamin C, vitamin E, beta-carotene

- 1 tablespoon light sesame or peanut oil
- 7 ounces (200 g) firm tofu, cut into chunks
- ¼ cup (50 g) baby corn
- ⅔ cup (100 g) snow peas, stringed
- 2 medium carrots, peeled and cut into julienne strips
- 2 cups (150 g) small broccoli florets
- 1 cup (100 g) shredded bok choy
- 1 cup (100 g) fresh bean sprouts
- 4 green onions, cut into 1-inch pieces
- 1 quarter-size piece fresh ginger, chopped
- 1 teaspoon Chinese five-spice powder

- 2 tablespoons reduced-sodium soy sauce
- ½ cup (125 ml) vegetable broth
- 2 teaspoons cornstarch

Heat the oil in a wok or large nonstick skillet and stir-fry the tofu until lightly golden. Add the corn, snow peas, carrots, and broccoli and stir-fry for 3 minutes. Add the bok-choy, bean sprouts, green onions, ginger, and five-spice powder and stir-fry for 2 minutes longer, adding a little soy sauce and a little vegetable broth as the pan gets dry.

Combine the remaining vegetable broth with the cornstarch and remaining soy sauce and add to the pan, stirring until the sauce thickens.

GOULASH OF WINTER VEGETABLES AND BEANS ✳

230 calories; 6g fat per serving

good source of
fiber, beta-carotene, vitamin C

- 1 tablespoon sunflower or canola oil
- 2 medium onions, peeled and sliced
- 3 medium carrots, peeled and chopped
- 4 medium celery stalks, chopped
- 1 tablespoon Hungarian paprika (or use Spanish paprika with a pinch of cayenne)
- 1 large potato, cubed
- 1 medium parsnip, peeled and cubed
- ⅔ cup (100 g) peeled and diced sweet potato
- 1 can (14 ounces/400 g) peeled tomatoes with juice
- ⅔ cup (150 g) canned red kidney beans
- 1 tablespoon tomato paste
- 2 teaspoons Italian seasoning
- 1¾ cups (400 ml) vegetable broth
- pinch each *salt and black pepper*
- ¼ cup (3 tablespoons) reduced-fat sour cream

Heat the oil in a large flameproof casserole and soften the onion in it for a few minutes. Stir in the carrots and celery. Cook for 5 minutes.

Add the paprika, stir for 1 minute, then add the rest of the ingredients except the sour cream, and stir well. Bring to a boil, reduce the heat, and simmer for 1 hour, or until everything is tender and a rich sauce forms.

Adjust the seasoning and dollop each serving with 1 tablespoon sour cream.

✳ *Undercook slightly if freezing.*

SPICED SALMON FISH CAKES WITH A CREAMED CAPER SAUCE *

280 calories; 13g fat per serving

good source of
omega-3 oils, vitamin E,
vitamin B6, protein

- *12 ounces (350 g) salmon fillet, lightly poached, microwaved, or baked; flaked*
- *12 ounces (350 g) russet baking pota toes, boiled until just tender, then peeled and coarsely mashed with dash hot-pepper sauce*
- *1 teaspoon chopped fresh or freeze-dried lemongrass (optional)*
- *juice of 1 small lime*
- *1 tablespoon chopped fresh cilantro leaves*
- *pinch ground ginger*
- *1 small red bell pepper, seeded, finely chopped, and steamed or microwaved for 1 minute, until just tender-crisp*
- *pinch each salt and black pepper*
- *1 egg and 1 egg yolk, beaten*

for the sauce:
- *⅓ cup (4 tablespoons) low-fat plain yogurt*
- *1 tablespoon reduced-fat sour cream*
- *1 tablespoon chopped well-drained capers*

In a bowl, combine all the fish cake ingredients except the eggs with a fork, making sure to leave at least some visible pieces of salmon. Add the beaten egg, mixing gently.

Form the mixture into 8 small patties (they will be pretty soft, but don't worry) and place on a lightly oiled baking sheet. Either bake for 20 minutes in a preheated 350°F oven or broil for 10 minutes, turning once, or until cakes are lightly golden and heated through.

Meanwhile, combine the sauce ingredients. Serve the fish cakes with the sauce.

❋ *Fish cakes will freeze; sauce won't.*

WHOLE FISH, CATALAN STYLE *

250 calories; 9g fat per portion

good source of
calcium, protein,
beta-carotene, vitamin C

- *1 tablespoon olive oil*
- *1 large Spanish onion, finely chopped*
- *1 large green bell pepper, seeded and coarsely chopped*
- *2 garlic cloves, minced*
- *1 can (14 ounces/400 g) crushed tomatoes*
- *¼ cup (4 tablespoons) strained chopped tomatoes*
- *1 tablespoon tomato paste*
- *pinch brown sugar*
- *16 black olives, pitted*
- *1 teaspoon each coarsely chopped fresh rosemary, basil, thyme*
- *pinch each salt and black pepper*
- *Four 5-ounce (150-g) red-snapper fillets*

Heat the oil in a large saucepan and sauté the onion and green bell pepper until soft and just golden. Add the garlic and cook for 1 or 2 minutes. Add the rest of the ingredients except the fish and simmer for 30 minutes until a rich sauce forms.

About 10 minutes from the end of cooking time, broil the fish for 6 to 8 minutes, until it is just opaque in the thickest part.

Serve the fish with the sauce.

Note: *This sauce recipe makes a good basic tomato sauce if you omit the green pepper and olives.*

❋ *Freeze sauce only; do not freeze fish.*

CHILI CHICKEN *

255 calories, 13g fat per serving

good source of
protein, vitamins C and E, beta-carotene

- *1 tablespoon sunflower or corn oil*
- *1 medium red onion, sliced*
- *1 pound (450 g) skinless, boneless chicken breast halves, cut into strips*
- *1 large red bell pepper, seeded and sliced*
- *2 teaspoons jerk or Cajun seasoning (more or less to taste, see Variation)*
- *1 medium zucchini, thinly sliced*
- *2 rings fresh pineapple (or canned in juice), cubed*
- *1 small ripe avocado, peeled, pitted, and chopped (do this just before cooking, or the avocado will discolor)*

Heat the oil in a large heavy nonstick skillet or wok and stir-fry the onion and chicken over medium to high heat until the chicken is golden and the onion partly cooked, about 3 minutes.

Reduce the heat slightly, add the bell pepper and jerk or Cajun seasoning and stir-fry for 2 to 3 minutes, until fragrant. Add the zucchini and pineapple and stir-fry for another minute, or until the zucchini is tender. Add the avocado, stir and serve.

Variation: *For a milder dish, add a pinch allspice instead of the jerk or Cajun seasoning.*

❋ *Freeze without the avocado. Add avocado when reheating.*

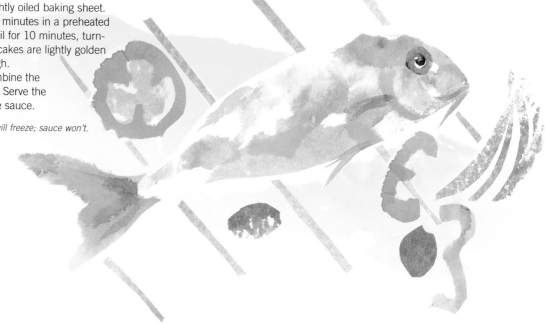

CHICKEN, LIME, AND MANGO BROCHETTES WITH A MINT RAITA SAUCE *

230 calories; 9g fat per serving

good source of
protein, magnesium, B vitamins, beta-carotene, vitamin C

- 3 limes, cut into quarters
- 1 garlic clove, minced
- 1 quarter-size piece fresh ginger, minced
- 2 tablespoons sunflower or canola oil
- 2 teaspoons honey
- 2 tablespoons reduced-sodium soy sauce
- pinch each salt and black pepper
- Four 4-5-ounce (100-150 g) skinless, boneless chicken breast halves, cubed
- 1 ripe mango

for the mint raita:
- 1/3 cup (4 tablespoons) low-fat plain yogurt
- 1 tablespoon chopped fresh mint

Several hours before you plan to eat, marinate the chicken. Grate the rind of one of the limes and reserve. Juice 2 of the limes and place into a glass dish. Add the lime rind, garlic, ginger, oil, honey, soy sauce, salt, and pepper to the dish and combine well with a wooden spoon. Add the chicken pieces and toss them in the marinade. Cover and let marinate in the refrigerator for up to 12 hours.

When ready to cook, peel and cube the mango and thread it with the chicken onto skewers. Arrange on a jelly-roll pan and broil, turning once, for about 4 minutes per side, basting with any remaining marinade once or twice.

Meanwhile, combine the yogurt and the mint to make the raita.

When the brochettes are cooked, serve them with any pan juices, the lime quarters, and the raita.

* Brochettes can be frozen cooked or uncooked. Sauce will not freeze.

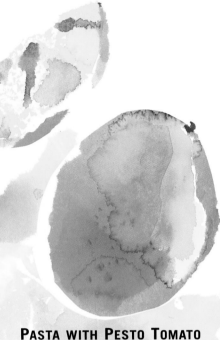

PASTA WITH PESTO TOMATO SAUCE *

425 calories; 22g fat per serving

good source of
calcium, vitamin C, vitamin E, and beta-carotene

- 1 small bunch fresh basil, stems removed
- 2 large garlic cloves, peeled
- 1/3 cup (50 g) grated fresh Parmesan cheese
- 2 tablespoons pine nuts
- pinch salt
- 4 medium-ripe large tomatoes, peeled, seeded, and diced
- 1/4 cup olive oil
- 10 ounces (275 g) pappardelle or fettuccini pasta

In a food processor, process the basil, garlic, Parmesan, pine nuts, and salt until finely chopped. Add the tomatoes and pulse just to mix. Drizzle the oil over the top of the sauce but do not mix in.

Cook the pasta until al dente in a large pot of lightly salted boiling water, about 10 minutes. Serve the sauce poured over the piping-hot drained pasta.

* You can freeze the sauce fairly successfully, or it will keep in an airtight container for a week or more in the refrigerator.

PASTA PRIMAVERA

450 calories; 9.5g fat per serving

good source of
fiber, vitamin C, calcium, and beta-carotene

- 11 ounces (300 g) pasta twists or penne
- 2/3 cup (150 g) frozen lima beans
- 4 small zucchini, sliced
- 1½ cups (200 g) baby carrots
- 8 tender asparagus tips
- 1/4 cup (50 g) fresh or frozen baby peas
- 4 baby leeks or large green onions, halved lengthwise and each half cut in half again
- 8 green onions, cut into 1-inch (2.5 cm) lengths
- 1 tablespoon olive oil
- 1/2 cup (100 ml) reduced-fat sour cream
- 1/4 cup (50 g) reduced-fat cottage cheese
- 1/4 cup (50 ml) skim milk
- 1/3 cup (50 g) grated fresh Parmesan cheese
- 2 teaspoons Dijon mustard
- pinch each salt and black pepper
- 2 tablespoons chopped fresh parsley, to garnish

Put a saucepan of lightly salted water on to boil for the pasta.

Parboil the lima beans, zucchini, and carrots in another pan of lightly salted water for 2 minutes and drain thoroughly.

Put the pasta in the boiling pasta water. Meanwhile, put the asparagus, peas, and leeks in a steamer set over a saucepan of boiling water. Steam for a few minutes until just tender.

While the pasta is boiling and the vegetables are steaming, heat the olive oil in a nonstick skillet. Sauté the lima beans, zucchini, carrots, and green onions in the olive oil over medium heat until slightly golden, but still with some bite (a few minutes), stirring once or twice.

Combine the sour cream, cottage cheese, skim milk, Parmesan, mustard, salt, and pepper in a small bowl. When the pasta is cooked, about 10 minutes, drain and toss with the steamed vegetables, the sautéed vegetables, and the sauce.

Garnish with the parsley to serve.

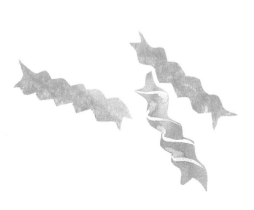

T his simple tone, strength, and stretch program devised and demonstrated by top personal trainer, Louise Taylor, RSA, will help you recover a more youthful shape and body definition. It lets you work hardest on the areas of your body that are most in need of attention. NOTE Always check with your doctor before beginning this or any exercise program, especially if you have arthritis or any medical condition that you think may prevent you from exercising, or if you have not done any exercise at all recently (see Rejuvenating Joints, page 51).

WORKSHOP **3** SHAPEWISE 1–TOTAL TONE

Before You Begin

Please read these notes and follow all the advice carefully every time you exercise. Bodies unaccustomed to exercise need nurturing, not punishing. It is very important always to exercise within your capabilities.

The basic T O T A L   T O N E program consists of a three-minute **W A R M - U P**, followed by five short **W A R M - U P   S T R E T C H E S**, then ten minutes of nine **T O T A L   T O N E   E X E R C I S E S**, followed by two to three minutes of **C O O L - D O W N   S T R E T C H E S**, which will also help your flexibility and posture.

This will give you a 20-minute workout. Don't exercise immediately after eating, or when ill or very tired.
A stamina–building aerobic program is detailed in Workshop 14.

D on't skip any of the exercises, in this section particularly the warm–up and stretches. If you don't warm up and cool down properly, you'll find the Total Tone exercises harder to do, and you will likely suffer muscular aches the next day.
• Run through the program slowly at first and pay close attention to the posture instructions and concentrate on the muscle(s) you are training. It's better to do an exercise well once than eight repeats "reps" incorrectly. Don't expect an underused body to cope with all the moves perfectly at first. You may not be able to achieve the same degree of stretch Louise achieves in the photos, or be able to hold an identical "finish" position in all of the exercises, but you will see and feel improvement week by week as long as you keep trying your very best.
• The Total Tone program is to be done three times a week (see the weekly schedules on pages 9–18) with rest days in between. Don't do your three sessions three days in a row; space them out evenly during the week. Your body needs a chance to recover and adapt. After you've been doing the program for two weeks, you may want to add another session or one of the optional Add-Ons to your workout.
• In addition to the basic Total Tone program, there are four short optional sections if you want to do extra work on your problem areas. After using the shape assessment results on page 21, add those sections you want to do to your session *after* the basic Total Tone Exercises but *before* the cool-down stretches. Don't attempt this extra work until you have been doing the basic program for at least two weeks and can do it well.
• Wear comfortable clothing, such as a T-shirt and shorts or a leotard and tights. Cold muscles are susceptible to injury. Until you are thoroughly warmed up, wear extra layers like a sweat suit and use it to keep warm during the cool-down stretches.

TIME TO WARM UP . . .

Allow three minutes to warm up all your major muscles. Take deep, even breaths throughout, and work up to a good momentum, with a smooth rhythm.

1 Start by marching in step. Tummy tucked in, head high, shoulders back but relaxed and down, march with arms swinging gently, gradually lifting your legs a little higher and arms pumping a little harder. March for about 30 seconds.

2 Move on to "step touches." Take a big step to the right with your right foot, then bring your left foot to meet it. Take a high step to the left and bring your right foot to meet the left. As you do so, begin circling your arms–first small circles, then larger ones. Step-touch for 30 seconds. Continue step-touching, but now punch your arms (fists closed) up toward the ceiling and back down. Step-touch and reach for 30 seconds.

3 Next, do double step-touches. Take one step to the right, bring your left foot to join the right, then take one more step to the right. Repeat to the left side. Move lightly across the floor, making the middle step into a small hop. As you step, lift your arms out straight to the sides and up, then bring them back down again. Do double step-touches for 30 seconds. By now you should be quite warm.

4 Do 30 seconds of hamstring curls. With feet hip-width apart, bring your right heel up behind you, bending the right knee. Feel the back of your right thigh working. Return foot to the floor and curl the left leg. Keep curling alternate legs and, as you do each curl, swing your arms up in front of you.

5 Finish with 30 seconds of "toe taps." With feet just over hip-width apart and weight on the left leg, point and tap the right toe out to the side; lightly transfer weight onto the right leg and repeat with the left toe. Repeat these taps and, as you do so, lift your arms alternately to reach overhead. Now you are warm. If you aren't, do the warm-up again, putting plenty of effort into it.

WARM-UP STRETCHES

Hold each for a count of 8 and breathe normally.

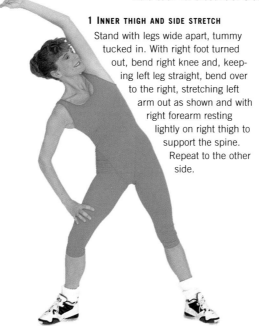

1 INNER THIGH AND SIDE STRETCH
Stand with legs wide apart, tummy tucked in. With right foot turned out, bend right knee and, keeping left leg straight, bend over to the right, stretching left arm out as shown and with right forearm resting lightly on right thigh to support the spine. Repeat to the other side.

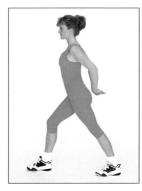

2 CALF AND CHEST STRETCH
Stand as shown, tummy tucked in, with left leg back and right knee bent, keeping body weight slightly forward. Clasp hands behind back and push the chest forward. Feel the stretch in your right calf and across your chest. Repeat with the other leg.

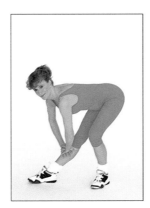

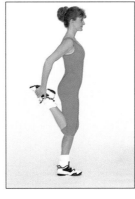

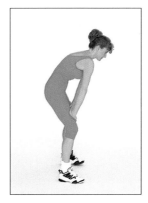

3 HAMSTRING (BACK OF THIGH) STRETCH
Stand as shown, with left leg behind right and left knee bent. Keeping right leg straight, bend over right leg and lift buttocks high, placing hands below right knee for support, until you feel a stretch in right hamstring. Repeat to other side.

4 STANDING QUADRICEPS (FRONT THIGH) STRETCH
Stand, tummy tucked in, feet hip-width apart, well balanced. Raise right foot behind you as shown and clasp foot, using right hand. Bring heel in to touch buttocks. Slowly release and repeat to the other side.

5 BACK STRETCH
Stand with feet hip-width apart, tummy tucked in and hands resting halfway down thighs. Curl your back into the letter "C," pulling tummy in toward spine as you do, then relax. Repeat four times in a slow and controlled manner. *Your warm-up is finished.*

THE TOTAL TONE EXERCISES

A Note about Repetitions

Over a few sessions increase the number of reps for each exercise until you can do the recommended number. If you are not used to exercising, you may find you can only do a few reps at the beginning, but you will soon get stronger. Work to the point where the muscle being trained tells you it has done enough (a slight trembling in the muscle is a good indication), do one more, then move onto the next exercise. Stop for a few seconds after each set of eight reps, if you like. Breathe normally throughout unless otherwise instructed. Once you have done the program several times at the full number of reps, you can add reps to increase your conditioning, stopping when your training muscle tells you it has done enough.

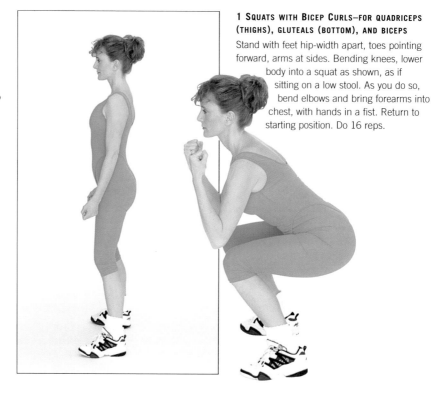

1 SQUATS WITH BICEP CURLS—FOR QUADRICEPS (THIGHS), GLUTEALS (BOTTOM), AND BICEPS

Stand with feet hip-width apart, toes pointing forward, arms at sides. Bending knees, lower body into a squat as shown, as if sitting on a low stool. As you do so, bend elbows and bring forearms into chest, with hands in a fist. Return to starting position. Do 16 reps.

2 PLIÉS WITH TRICEPS EXTENSIONS —FOR INNER THIGH AND TRICEPS (BACK OF UPPER ARMS)

Stand with legs wide apart, toes pointing outward, arms at sides as shown. Keeping feet flat on the floor, chest up, and tummy tucked in, bend at the knees and lower your body until your thighs are parallel to the floor (or as low as you can get). As you do so, bring your arms straight out behind you as shown, keeping shoulders relaxed and palms facing inward. Return to starting position. Do 16 reps.

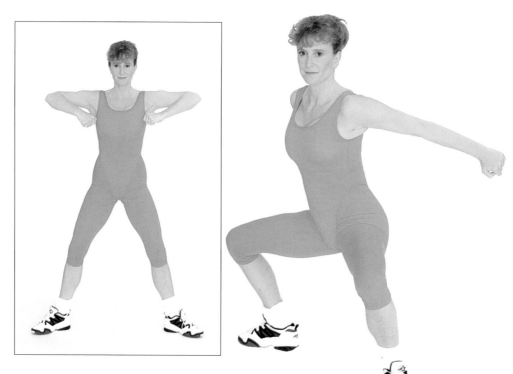

**3 FORWARD LUNGES WITH PECTORAL FLIES
—FOR QUADRICEPS, HAMSTRINGS, GLUTEALS,
AND PECTORALS (CHEST)**
Stand with feet hip-width apart and arms raised at sides as shown. Take a big step forward on your right leg, bending both knees to 90°. Keep your right knee over your heel and lift left heel off floor. As you do, bring elbows and forearms to meet in front of your chest. Return to starting position for arms and legs, repeat with left leg and both arms. Do 8 reps on each leg, alternately.

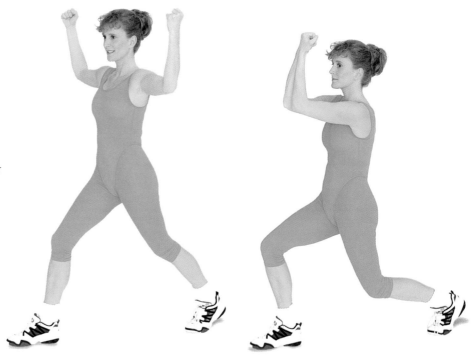

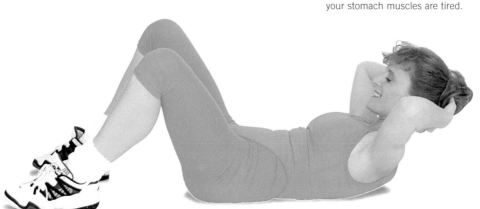

**4 ABDOMINAL CRUNCHES—FOR
ABDOMINALS (STOMACH)**
Lie on your back on a mat or towel, fingers lightly placed behind head, knees bent, feet flat on floor and tummy pulled in as shown. Breathing out, lift your head and tops of shoulders off the floor, using your stomach muscles to bring you up, NOT your hands or neck. Keep your chin off your chest. Keep the movement controlled. Slowly lower. Do 16 reps. If your neck begins to ache, stop–this means your stomach muscles are tired.

EXERCISE PROFILE

Sue
By the end of week 4, Sue has lost 2 inches off her hips and 1½ inches off her waist, and was really enjoying her exercises. Her stamina is already excellent and, she says, "I feel better and more full of energy."

EXERCISE PROFILE

Pamela has always disliked any kind of formal exercise, and, at 57, found it very challenging to begin a toning program coupled with an aerobic regimen.

"At first I couldn't do more than one or two of the toning repeats and could do no more than a few minutes' aerobic exercise at a time."

By Week 8, however, Pam was up to par in both areas, and more supple–an important point for her. She had also lost 3 inches off her waist.

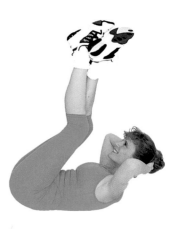

5 DIAGONAL CRUNCHES–FOR WAIST

In the same starting position as for abdominal crunches (page 39), come up again, but this time bring your right arm and shoulder across toward your left knee, slowly lower, then bring your left shoulder up toward your right knee. Lower and do 16 reps on each side, alternately.

6 DOUBLE CRUNCHES–FOR ABDOMINALS

Same starting position as for abdominal crunches (page 39). Raise legs in air as shown, with ankles crossed and knees slightly bent. Come up as in the abdominal crunches, but this time try to lift your buttocks off the floor at the same time raising your shoulders. Pause, then release to the floor. Breathe out as you lift and keep your chin lifted; inhale as you lower. Do 8 reps.

7 SIDE LEG RAISES–FOR HIPS AND OUTER THIGHS

Turn onto your left side and lie as shown, with your left leg bent, right leg straight but knee relaxed. Keeping hips aligned (don't allow right hip to slip back, or the exercise will be less effective), slowly lift right leg (not too high), leading with your heel. Lower slowly. Keep buttocks tightly clenched throughout. Do 32 reps, then turn over and do 32 reps on the other side.

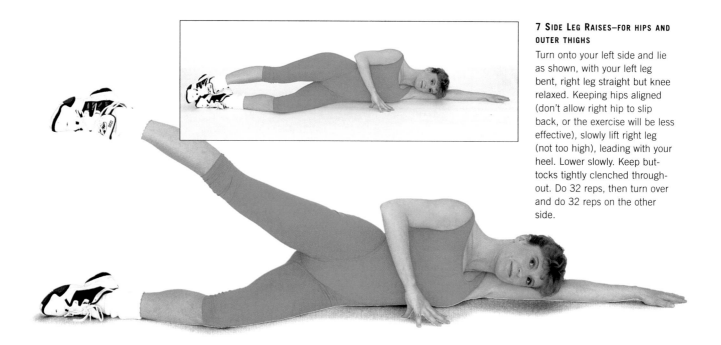

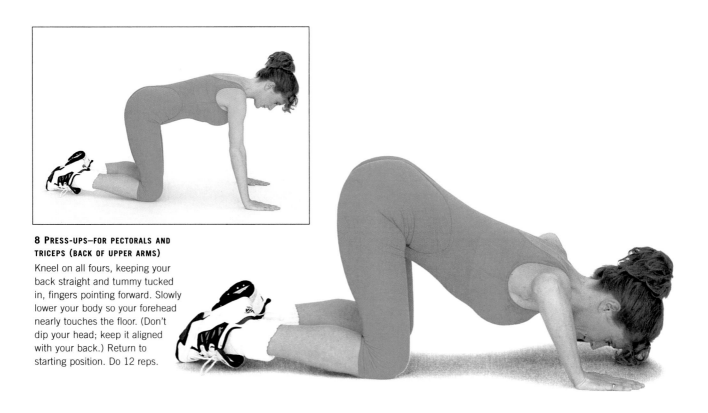

8 Press-ups—for pectorals and triceps (back of upper arms)

Kneel on all fours, keeping your back straight and tummy tucked in, fingers pointing forward. Slowly lower your body so your forehead nearly touches the floor. (Don't dip your head; keep it aligned with your back.) Return to starting position. Do 12 reps.

9 Back extensions—for lower back

Lie face down on floor, resting your head on your hands as shown. Lift your upper body and arms a few inches off the floor. Don't use your feet as a pivot while doing this; use your back muscles. Always look at the floor. Slowly return to starting position. Do 12 reps.

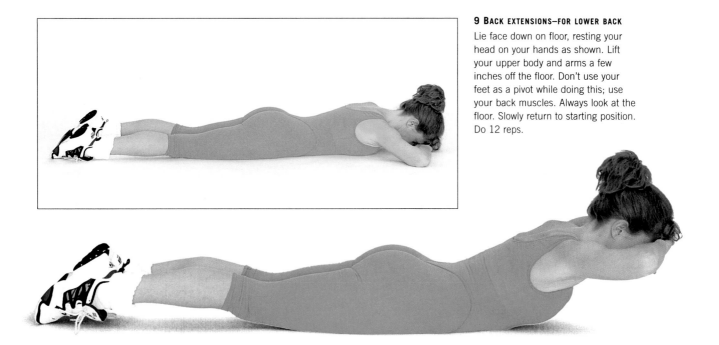

COOL-DOWN STRETCHES

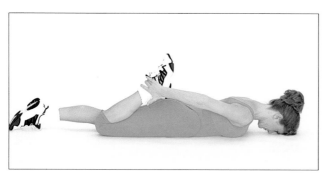

1 QUADRICEPS STRETCH

Lie face down, arms at sides. Bend your right knee and bring your right foot in toward your buttocks. Hold your right foot with your right hand and gently pull your foot a little further down, to feel a good stretch along the front of your right thigh. Hold for a count of 8, relax, and repeat to other side.

2 CALF STRETCH

Turn over and lie on your back, knees bent, feet on floor. Lift your right leg into the air as shown and flex your foot as hard as you can, trying to get your toes pointing as far down toward your head as possible. Feel a stretch along your right calf. Hold for a count of 12. Bring leg down to starting position and repeat the stretch with left leg.

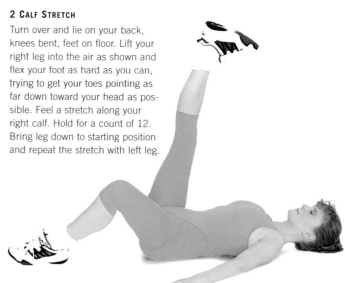

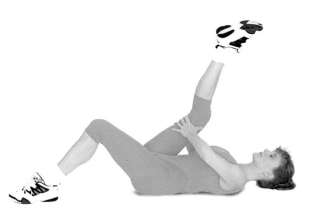

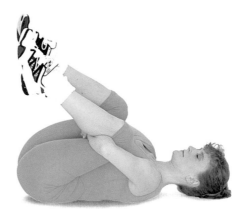

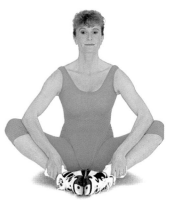

3 HAMSTRING STRETCH

In the same starting position as for the previous exercises, bring your right leg in toward your chest, clasping your hand behind your thigh as shown and straightening your leg as much as possible. Feel the stretch all along the back of your right thigh. Hold for a count of 16, trying to straighten the leg a little more toward the end of the stretch. Return to starting position and repeat with the other leg.

4 LOWER BACK STRETCH

From the same starting position as for the previous two exercises, slowly bring your knees in to your chest, using your hands to pull them in a little further. Feel a stretch in your lower back. Hold for a count of 12.

5 INNER THIGH STRETCH

Sit up and place the soles of your feet together in front of you. Keeping your lower back straight (don't slump), place hands on ankles as shown and gently push both thighs down toward the floor with your elbows until you feel a stretch along both inner thighs. Hold for a count of 12.

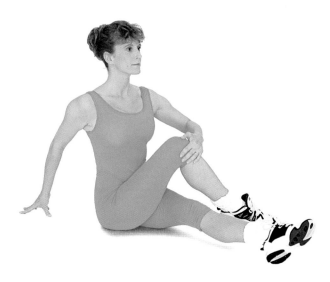

6 GLUTEAL STRETCH

Still sitting, with left leg straight on the floor, bring right foot over left leg and place it on the floor near your left hip. With your left hand, gently press the knee toward your chest. Feel the stretch in right buttock muscle. Hold for a count of 8. Repeat to other side.

7 CHEST STRETCH

Still sitting, with legs in a comfortable position in front of you, clasp your hands behind your back, palms facing outward, and pull your arms out away from your body. Feel a stretch across your chest. Hold for a count of 8.

10 SIDE STRETCH

Still sitting, place your right hand on the floor and bring your left arm up toward the ceiling and over your head, leaning over to the right slightly as you do so. Feel a stretch all along your left side. Hold for a count of 8 and repeat to the other side.

That completes your basic Total Tone Exercises. Don't forget to add on any of the following exercises for your particular "trouble spots" if you like–they should be done BEFORE the cool-down stretches.

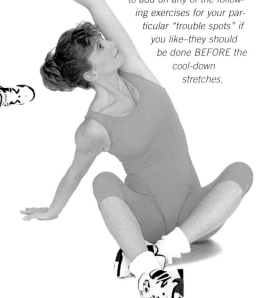

8 TRICEP STRETCH

Sitting in the same position as for the previous stretch, raise your right arm above your head and bend your elbow, putting your hand and palm inward, in the center of your upper back. Using your left hand behind your right elbow, press your right arm back to feel a stretch along your tricep (back of upper arm). Hold for a count of 8. Return to starting position and repeat with left arm.

9 UPPER BACK STRETCH

Still in the same sitting position, bring your arms out in front of you and clasp your fingers and palms outward. Push your hands away from your body until you feel a stretch across your upper back. Hold for a count of 8.

ADD-ONS. . . ADD-ONS. . . ADD-ONS. . .

Waist and Stomach

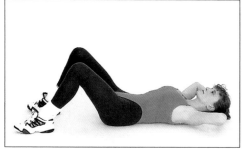

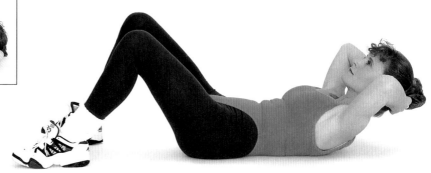

PULSING CRUNCHES

Lie on your back with knees bent, feet flat on floor, fingers loosely clasped behind head, elbows wide. Pull your stomach in toward floor and, using abdominal muscles, lift head and upper back off floor as shown. Instead of returning to the floor as in the basic crunches on page 39, return just halfway to the floor before coming up again. Repeat 16 times. Make these pulsing movements faster than ordinary crunches. *And remember–your head doesn't touch the floor until you've finished your reps!*

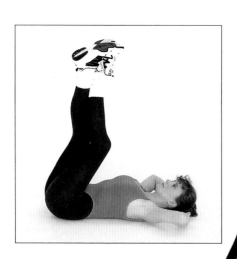

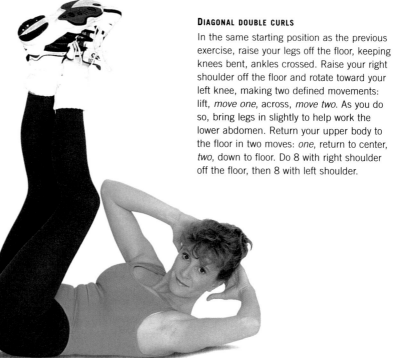

DIAGONAL DOUBLE CURLS

In the same starting position as the previous exercise, raise your legs off the floor, keeping knees bent, ankles crossed. Raise your right shoulder off the floor and rotate toward your left knee, making two defined movements: lift, *move one*, across, *move two*. As you do so, bring legs in slightly to help work the lower abdomen. Return your upper body to the floor in two moves: *one*, return to center, *two*, down to floor. Do 8 with right shoulder off the floor, then 8 with left shoulder.

Hips and Thighs

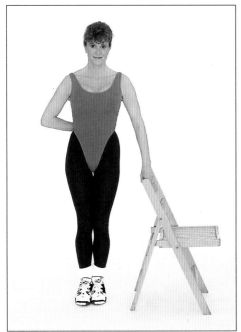
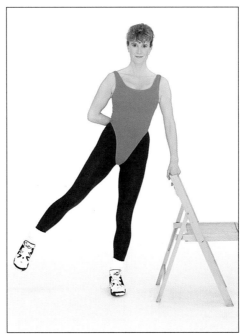

STANDING SIDE LEG RAISES

Stand with left side facing the back of a sturdy chair, feet hip-width apart and left hand holding chair back for support. Keeping leg straight but knee relaxed, slowly raise your right leg out to the side until you feel the right hip working. Hold for a count of 2, then slowly return to starting position. Do 8 reps, then repeat 8 on other side.

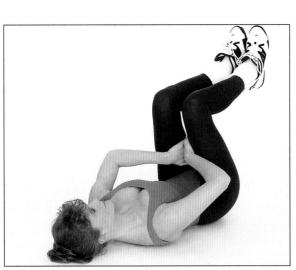

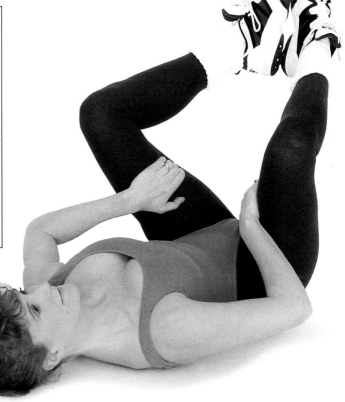

FROG'S-LEG PRESS

Lie on your back with feet together in the air as shown. Place hands on inner thighs and let knees drop open. Now try to bring knees back together while pressing down with your hands. Return to the starting position. Keep tummy pulled in throughout. Do 16 reps.

Buttocks and Hamstrings

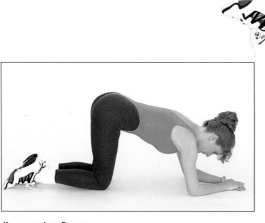

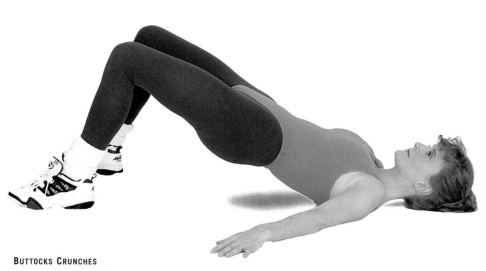

KNEELING LEG RAISES

Kneel on a mat, resting upper body on forearms and keeping tummy pulled in and back straight. Extend right leg off floor to lifted straight position as shown, until you feel your right gluteal muscle working, and return to starting position. Don't swing the leg, and only lift as high as you need to feel the buttock contract. Do 16 reps, then repeat with left leg.

BUTTOCKS CRUNCHES

Lie on your back with knees slightly bent, arms out at your sides, and feet flat on the floor. Use your gluteals to raise your pelvis off the floor as far as you can, still keeping your feet flat on the floor. Lower slowly and do 32 reps. Concentrate on pulling your gluteal muscles in tight to achieve this.

EXERCISE PROFILE

Kay was very uncoordinated in her movements at the start of the program and very weak and lacking in confidence in her own ability to improve. She persisted, however, and toward the end of the ten weeks, her body shape, fitness level, and muscle tone improved so much that even we were surprised! "One of the reasons I gave up smoking was that exercise and cigarettes don't go together. I want healthy lungs now. And I find that regular exercise actually removes the craving for cigarettes, anyway!"

Chest and Upper Arms

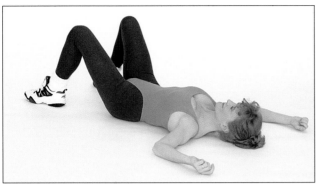

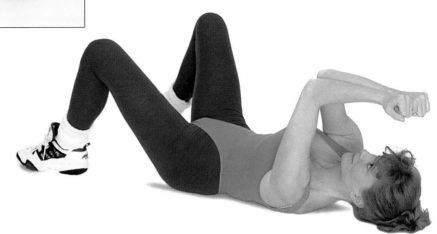

LYING CHEST PRESS

Lie on your back with knees bent, feet flat on floor, tummy tucked in, and arms out to each side as shown. With fists closed, bring arms in together until elbows and forearms meet above your chest as shown. Feel your chest and arm muscles working. Lower to starting position and do 16 reps. You can use light weights for this exercise in later weeks.

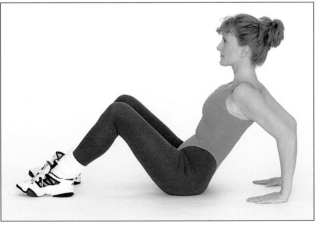

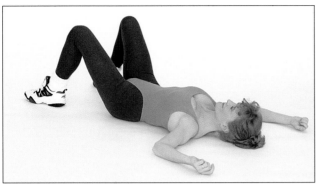

TRICEP DIPS

Sit on the floor with knees bent and arms slightly behind you on each side, with fingers pointing forward, as shown. Bend elbows and slowly lower upper body toward the floor to about 45°. Slowly return to starting position. Do 16 reps.

Y *ou can lose several years, several pounds, and several inches in seconds*
just by the way you stand. So here's where you check your body
alignment. Good body-alignment–posture is as important to the shape
and look of your body as are being a reasonable weight and being well toned.

SHAPEWISE 2–BODY ALIGNMENT

It is a sad fact that by the time they hit their middle years–and often long before then–nine out of ten women have very poor posture, adding years to the way they look. Double chins and a protruding stomach are as likely to be caused by pelvic, hip, and spine misalignment as by fat. A thick waist isn't just "middle-aged spread," but a result of years spent sitting incorrectly in office, dining, and easy chairs. However, if you relearn how to sit, stand, and walk correctly, with straight shoulders, long neck, and pelvis slightly tilted forward, these problems will be minimized, or even disappear, in time.

Viewed from the side, you can seem to shed pounds just by aligning your body (see photos at right). And there are other benefits to standing tall, as well. Good posture gives you authority, helps you to look confident, outgoing, and in control. People will view you as a more positive person and you will feel so yourself. You will also appear more youthful, as poor posture is associated with old age. Back pain, which plagues most of us at least sometimes, will also be minimized.

Although it is possible to realign your body in front of a mirror almost instantly, the improvements you make will need to be reinforced by doing regular body-alignment exercises until that posture has become completely natural to you. Without this, you may be able to hold the correct position for a minute or two, but your muscles will quickly tire. That is because years of misalignment have caused certain muscles to shorten and tighten, others to

The Pelvic Tilt

The core of good posture is getting your pelvis into correct alignment, so the first thing to do is practice the pelvic tilt several times a day until it becomes natural to you. Practice by tilting the top of your pelvis first forward (photo 1), then backward (photo 3), and finally center it so that your body is in correct centered alignment (photo 2).

When you are centered correctly, you should have your shoulders relaxed and down, your knees relaxed, your stomach should flatten out, and you should feel the base of your spine under your buttocks, which will be contracted slightly. Your lower back will flatten out (Louise has a pronounced lower back curve naturally; yours may be flatter). You should also feel your ribcage expand slightly, and your chin should be parallel to the floor.

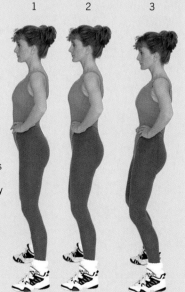

This pelvic position should be maintained when you are sitting, walking, or lying in bed, and when exercising. Get in the habit of thinking about this correct alignment throughout the day and eventually, with the help of the exercises in this section to retrain your muscles, it will become second nature.

lengthen and weaken. You have to exercise to reverse this process and strengthen the muscles to work as they were meant to work.

As an example, if you have rounded shoulders, the muscles of your upper back and back of shoulders will have lengthened and weakened, while the opposite muscles of your chest and front shoulders will have shortened and tightened. To correct round shoulders permanently, you need to strengthen those weak muscles and stretch those short, tight ones. Only when you have done that will the correct posture feel natural to you.

The Total Tone program in Workshop 3 will help toward making these changes, but if your posture is really poor you will need extra work. In ten weeks you can achieve a lot, especially if you make a conscious effort all day, every day, to put correct alignment into practice. After all, a few minutes daily exercise won't help much if you spend the remaining hours of the day sitting, standing, walking and lying with bad posture. It is during this time you should practice doing everything right.

The exercise suggestions that comprise Workshop 4 are designed to help correct the most common posture faults that develop in the middle years (see right). If your figure problems seem to be different from those described here or, indeed, if you want more personal advice on your own body alignment problems, there are several internationally recognized systems with classes worldwide. Check out what you have available in your area. Your local library, YMCA, or the Internet can help you locate classes. For example, the Alexander Technique increases awareness of movement, posture, and balance in your daily life. Iyengar Yoga teaches total body awareness, breathing, and relaxation.

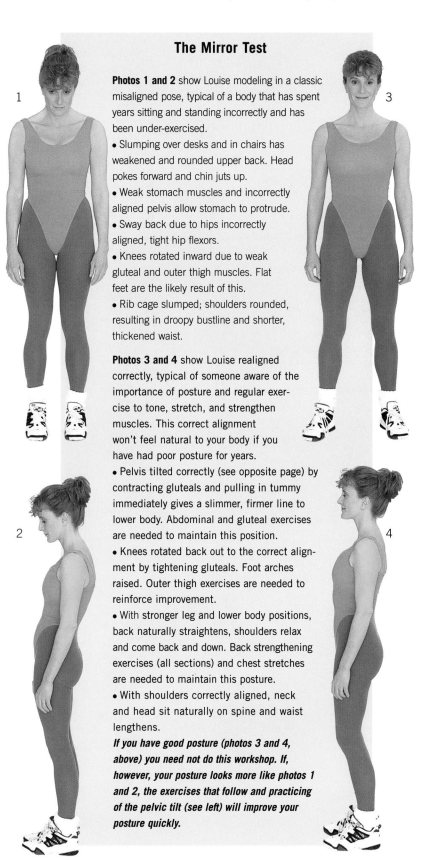

The Mirror Test

Photos 1 and 2 show Louise modeling in a classic misaligned pose, typical of a body that has spent years sitting and standing incorrectly and has been under-exercised.
- Slumping over desks and in chairs has weakened and rounded upper back. Head pokes forward and chin juts up.
- Weak stomach muscles and incorrectly aligned pelvis allow stomach to protrude.
- Sway back due to hips incorrectly aligned, tight hip flexors.
- Knees rotated inward due to weak gluteal and outer thigh muscles. Flat feet are the likely result of this.
- Rib cage slumped; shoulders rounded, resulting in droopy bustline and shorter, thickened waist.

Photos 3 and 4 show Louise realigned correctly, typical of someone aware of the importance of posture and regular exercise to tone, stretch, and strengthen muscles. This correct alignment won't feel natural to your body if you have had poor posture for years.
- Pelvis tilted correctly (see opposite page) by contracting gluteals and pulling in tummy immediately gives a slimmer, firmer line to lower body. Abdominal and gluteal exercises are needed to maintain this position.
- Knees rotated back out to the correct alignment by tightening gluteals. Foot arches raised. Outer thigh exercises are needed to reinforce improvement.
- With stronger leg and lower body positions, back naturally straightens, shoulders relax and come back and down. Back strengthening exercises (all sections) and chest stretches are needed to maintain this posture.
- With shoulders correctly aligned, neck and head sit naturally on spine and waist lengthens.

If you have good posture (photos 3 and 4, above) you need not do this workshop. If, however, your posture looks more like photos 1 and 2, the exercises that follow and practicing of the pelvic tilt (see left) will improve your posture quickly.

THE BODY ALIGNMENT EXERCISES

Do these exercises as often as you can. Add them to your Total Tone program or fit them in whenever you like. Always warm up before exercising and cool down afterward (if doing alignment exercises separately from the Total Tone program, use the Total Tone warm-up and cool-down stretches).

Abdominal strength

Do extra work on the Abdominal Crunches, Diagonal Crunches, and Double Crunches that appear on pages 39 and 40 in the basic Total Tone Exercises, plus the Add-Ons for Waist and Stomach (page 44).

Gluteal (buttock) strength

Do extra work on the Squats, Forward Lunges, and Side Leg Raises that appear on pages 38, 39, and 40 in the basic Total Tone Exercises, plus the Add-Ons for Buttocks and Hamstrings (page 46).

Back strength

Do extra work on the Back Extensions that appear on page 41 in the basic Total Tone Exercises, plus the two exercises pictured here.

Chest strength

Do extra work on the Calf and Chest Stretch described in the Total Tone Warm-Up (page 37), extra work on the Chest Stretch in the Total Tone Cool-Down (page 43), plus the three stretches described on the opposite page.

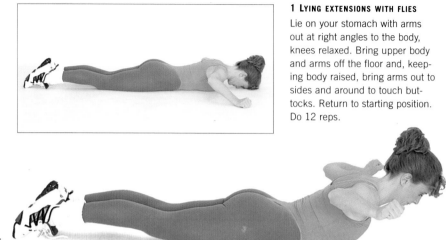

1 LYING EXTENSIONS WITH FLIES
Lie on your stomach with arms out at right angles to the body, knees relaxed. Bring upper body and arms off the floor and, keeping body raised, bring arms out to sides and around to touch buttocks. Return to starting position. Do 12 reps.

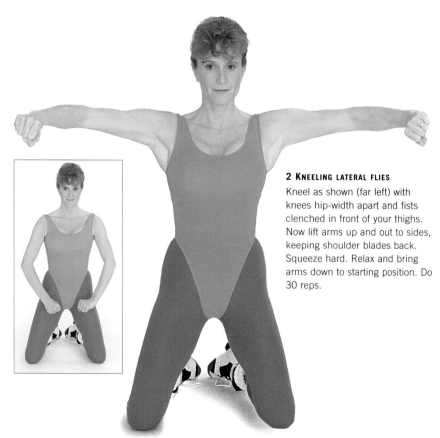

2 KNEELING LATERAL FLIES
Kneel as shown (far left) with knees hip-width apart and fists clenched in front of your thighs. Now lift arms up and out to sides, keeping shoulder blades back. Squeeze hard. Relax and bring arms down to starting position. Do 30 reps.

All-Day Tips

✔ Think about your body as often as you can. Get into the habit of correcting your posture all the time, even while driving.

✘ Don't sit with your legs crossed.

✘ Don't stand with your weight on one leg.

✘ Don't wear high heels all the time; they encourage poor posture and back-aches.

✔ Remember that posture faults that have developed over many years will take time to correct. Don't give up!

✔ Check your office, dining, and easy chairs for support. Many chairs are designed to encourage bad posture. Sit comfortably with your lower back supported by the back of the chair. If it is too deep, add firm cushions or pillows.

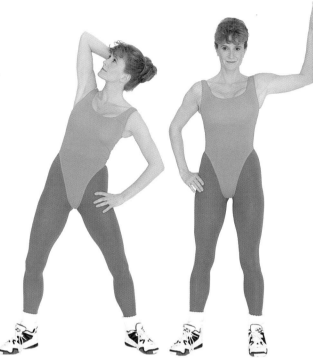

3 CHEST STRETCH 1

Stand as shown, left hand on left thigh, right hand behind head. Bend slightly to the left, keeping back aligned with hips. Feel the stretch in right side of chest as you move right elbow back. Hold and then relax. Repeat to other side.

4 CHEST STRETCH 2

Stand with your left side to a wall as shown, forearm and palm touching wall. Feel stretch across chest. Gently move chest forward (moving chest only) and feel stretch increase. Hold, then relax. Repeat to other side.

Rejuvenating Joints

Many people–even those as young as their mid-forties–have said to me, "It's too late for me to take up exercise. I feel too stiff and my joints won't take it." Osteoarthritis, the "wear and tear" type, can begin at any age, but is more common after the middle years. Most specialists agree that exercising is beneficial to arthritis sufferers (if it is gentle and done sensibly), and even more important, can help keep arthritis at bay.

Stretching exercises help mobility and toning exercises are as important to the arthritis sufferer as they are to anyone else–if not more so! If you have arthritis, your doctor should provide you with suitable exercises and/or refer you to a physiotherapist. He or she might recommend you begin with regular walking (with cushioned shoes and preferably on short grass.)

You could show him or her the Total Tone exercises in this book to see if they are suitable for you. The stretches that appear in the Total Tone program (warm-up and cool-down) might be suitable because you take the stretch just as far as you can and no further. But not all aches and pains are due to arthritis; they may well be simply the result of inactivity. If that is the case, check with your doctor that it is okay to exercise, then begin as soon as possible, taking things at your own pace.

You only have to look at the vast numbers of people of 50, 60, 70-plus at yoga classes, aquarobics, and so on, to realize there is no age at which you have to hang up your sneakers and say, "That's it–I'm too old." With common sense and motivation, you can improve your body and help yourself to feel and look better, whatever your age.

5 THE LONG BODY STRETCH

The long body stretch photographed here will help you achieve good overall body posture and is not quite as easy as it looks! Lie on your back on a mat, arms at sides, legs out straight. Squeeze gluteals, point toes. Elongate waist as far as you can (wiggle your bottom down the floor to achieve this), and raise arms up and over your head until backs of hands are touching the floor (you may not be able to do this, but go as far as you can without arching back). Feel your shoulder and rib cage stretching out, feel your stomach flattening into the floor, and breathe deeply and slowly. Hold the stretch for a count of 30, making sure you aren't raising your midsection off the floor to try to accommodate the stretch. As you get into the stretch you may find your hand reaching closer to the floor. Come up from the stretch gently by rolling on your side. In time you may want to hold this stretch for 2 to 3 minutes.

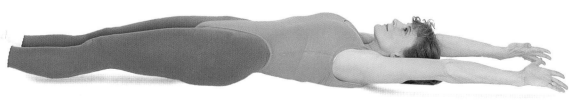

*M*ost of us think we look after our skin well, but few of us actually do, despite spending a fortune on face creams and cleansers. In this workshop, we sort out fact from fiction and get down to the bare essentials that really work to make your skin look, and feel, younger.

BARE ESSENTIALS

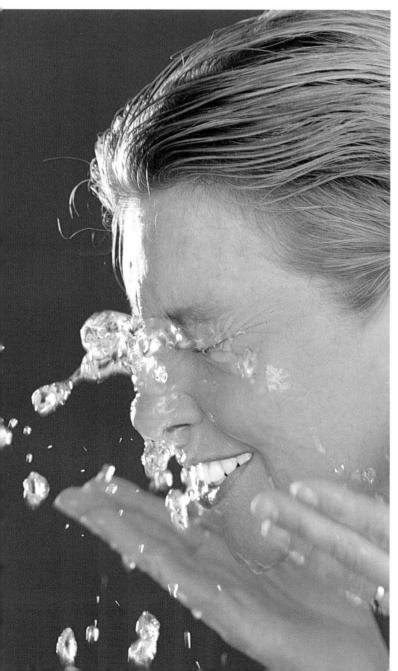

When we think of the aging face, we usually think first in terms of wrinkles, yet there are various other factors that also affect how old a face looks. Bags and sags, coarse skin texture, dull skin tone, dark shadows—all these can age you more than a few "expression lines." True, it is easier to prevent these problems than to cure them, nevertheless, you shouldn't think that the only way to rejuvenate your face is to schedule a surgical facelift. Other less drastic strategies can work almost as well as surgery.

War on wrinkles

Many factors can affect the amount, pattern, and depth of wrinkling, and most of these factors are things you can alter. Adopt as many of the following strategies as you can, both to delay onset of new wrinkles and to diminish the appearance of the wrinkles you already have.

● Moisturize regularly. Most women over 30 use a daytime moisturizer and a night cream, too—but most don't use them properly. To be effective, moisturizers need to be used every morning and night—generously. If you can't afford to liberally apply a product on your face and neck every single day, then don't buy an expensive cream. I've watched women "moisturize" their faces by putting a small dab of cream in the middle of each cheek then trying to spread it to the forehead, and around the eyes, and the chin; the very areas that need it most getting virtually none. Buy a cream you can lavish. (See box, "Which Cream is for You?," overleaf.)

If you buy nothing else, buy a daytime moisturizer that is absorbed quickly and can be used as a makeup base, and a heavier night cream or oil that gets a chance to work while you sleep. A separate eye cream is also a good idea, as these are formulated to be "light" and easy to apply to the delicate skin around your eyes, but this is not essential.

● Water your skin inside and out. Drinking lots of water–at least eight glasses a day–really does improve the skin's condition, and my own skin benefits very much from a morning spray of mineral water before moisturizing.

● Relax. A tense face encourages the formation of wrinkles, especially around the outer eyes, bridge of nose, and on the forehead. When people are sleeping peacefully they look much younger because in relaxed sleep all the expression lines are smoothed away. Similarly, if you are happy more often than you are miserable or angry, your face will reflect that as you get older. Laughter lines are fine, but frown lines or down lines are not flattering! If you find it hard to keep your face relaxed, get into the habit of regularly relaxing your jaw and unclenching your teeth, and destress the eye area by exerting shiatsu pressure with the middle fingers of each hand just on either side of the bridge of your nose, just below the eyebrows. Hold the pressure for 20 seconds. Do the same with fingers below the outer eye on the edge of the socket bone.

● Give up smoking and avoid smokey atmospheres. Smoking causes the capillaries to the skin to constrict, thereby preventing it from receiving the beneficial supply of oxygen and nutrients it needs to remain supple.

● Eat a diet high in antioxidants (such as the diet plans in this book), which "mop up" the free radicals.

The antioxidants are vitamins A, C, and E, and the mineral selenium.

● Keep your weight steady and don't get too thin. If your weight constantly yo-yoes more than seven pounds or so, it eventually shows on your face. Also, if you become too thin your face may lose its natural padding of fat, which helps to plump out lines. Lastly, don't lose weight too quickly or, again, wrinkles will be more likely to show.

● Keep the sun off your face. Contrary to most expert opinion, I'm a great believer in a little sun being good for the spirit and a great relaxer, but I *never* worship the sun with my face or body. I will sit out in the sun in very small doses during all seasons–very well protected by a sunscreen with a SPF factor of at least 15. Wear a high-factor sunscreen, good-quality sunglasses, and a brimmed hat, because the sun will damage the thin layers of skin on your face if you let it, destroying the collagen and elastin fibers of the dermis which encourages wrinkles and red spider veins. Both UVA and UVB rays are now known to cause premature skin aging and skin cancer. If you like the look of a tan, get a tube (many brands are now quite good) and keep the sun off your face.

● "Weather-beaten" is an expression that is very apt. Almost any kind of adverse weather will affect your skin, not just the sun. Protect your skin with moisturizer and hydrating makeup against the cold and winds. Check out the "weather" indoors, too–heating will dry out your skin and cause fine lines. If you can, take a mineral water spray to work and spray your face regularly if the atmosphere is dry, and moisturize once during the day.

The best weather for your face? Barely warm–and raining. So walking in the rain is not such a bad thing after all!

Stop the Drop

Although we worry so much about wrinkles, in fact, I don't believe they are the main enemy. It is the "sags and bags" on the face that are so aging, such as eyelids or brows that have dropped, eye bags, and jowly chins or jawlines that have lost their definition. The good news is you can do a great deal to "stop the drop."

Here's how:

● Maintain a reasonably consistent weight. Avoid "yo-yo" dieting or losing many pounds, which will cause the loose skin on your face to become a problem.

● Keep your face well exercised (*see "Exercise Your Face" box overleaf*). People rarely think about the muscles in their faces but, like the body muscles, they need regular toning workouts, too.

● Diminish eye bags with an eye pack twice a day. Cold used herbal tea bags, or slices of cucumber or raw potato placed on each closed eye for a few minutes will reduce puffiness considerably. You can also buy gels that have a similar effect and which you can apply under makeup.

Skin Condition

Skin texture, tone, and condition alter as we age. Here are some of the most common changes, with solutions.

Dryness

Dry, flaky, rough patches of skin should improve greatly with your antiwrinkle routine (page 52). If they still persist, try a mild facial scrub, but make sure it is very mild–labeled "for sensitive skin." Alternatively, two to three times a week rub a paste of oatmeal mixed with honey into your face, then rinse and moisturize. If your skin isn't sensitive, you can also use a mild moisturizer/night cream containing AHA. AHAs exfoliate the top layers of skin, revealing new skin underneath. However, I would never use an AHA cream every day–three or four times a week is plenty.

Open pores, blackheads

Far from just a plague of the teen years, open pores can actually get worse around the menopause. Pores need a tricky combination of deep cleansing with fairly gentle treatment. Contrary to what many experts say, skin toning lotions don't close open pores; they simply make the skin feel tauter by their astringent and/or cooling action. If you use a good light cleanser or facial wash, toner isn't necessary, especially if your skin is dry. Thorough rinsing with lukewarm water, or a spray of mineral water, tissued gently off, is all you need to remove any last traces of dirt and leave skin fresh.

Large, blocked pores respond best to three things: exercise, steaming (if you don't have acne or roacea), and masks. Your skin is an organ, and needs oxygen. To oxygenate it properly you need good circulation, which means regular aerobic exercise. By now you should be doing the Stamina program in Workshop 14, and should see improvements in your skin tone. Twice a week, put your cleansed face over a bowl of steaming hot water and keep it there for two minutes. Cleanse again and put on a refining face mask just over the open pored areas (see Face Masks, below). Wash off with lukewarm water after 15 minutes and moisturize.

Pallor

As skin gets older it tends to lose its pink tones and "fades." You can counteract this with enough sleep, a healthy diet containing plenty of vitamins and minerals, and plenty of exercise. Do all you can to improve the circulation to the face, including massage and facial exercises (see opposite page and the self-massage described on page 110). Lastly, as stress can cause pallor and dark undereye circles, try all the antistress treatments described in Workshop 15.

Eyes

I know your eyes aren't skin, but as healthy bright eyes can take years off your appearance, here are some tips for getting that bright-eyed look. You need enough sleep (but not too much), a diet rich in vitamin C, a life you enjoy (depression dulls the eyes), and every now and again, before a special occasion, use eye drops that clear the eye whites.

Face Masks

Try one of the many commercial masks available or make a natural food face mask to suit your skin. If you have combination skin, say, open pores around the nose or chin but dry elsewhere, put two different masks on at the same time. (Test a small area first, as some people have a reaction to food products on the skin.)

Enriching, moisturizing masks: mashed avocado, honey, and cream; mashed banana mixed with egg yolk; mayonnaise; honey and wheatgerm oil.

Refining masks for oily areas and coarse skin: egg white and oatmeal; egg white and lemon juice; kaolin, yogurt, and oatmeal.

Surgery-Free Face-Lift

Spend several minutes a day exercising the parts of your face
that seem most inclined to droop. Within a few weeks you'll notice a real
difference in your appearance as the muscles tone up
and your skin looks tauter.

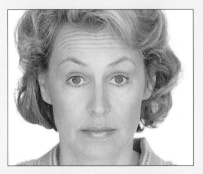

EYEBROW RAISE

Droopy brows make you look tired and
sad. Sit with face relaxed, including jaw
and teeth, and look straight ahead. Raise
eyebrows up as high as they will go while
keeping the rest of your face still. Hold the
raise for a count of 5, lower and repeat for
1 minute.

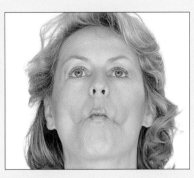

LOWER CHEEK SHAPER

Good if you have little cheek definition. Sit
as for the eyebrow raise, lift chin up and
out. Suck in your cheeks as tightly as you
can and hold for a count of 10. Relax and
repeat for 1 minute.

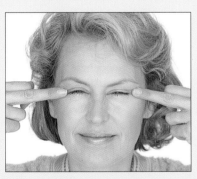

UPPER LID STRENGTHENER

Hooded lids "close up" your eyes, giving a
tired, aged look. Sit as above. Place middle
fingers of both hands on the outer edge of
both top lids (feel the bone at the edge of
the socket to locate). Keep a medium pressure with the fingers. Now squint lower lids
up hard and, as you do so, you'll feel a
strong muscle contraction under your
fingers. Do this small movement rapidly 10
times, relax for 1 minute, then repeat the
10 pulses plus the relax.

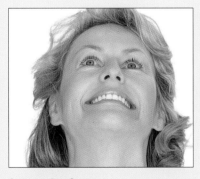

CHIN AND JAW SHAPER

For double chin, jowls, and saggy jawline.
Sit as above. Tilt head back and up slightly. Jut chin out slightly. Open mouth widely
by lowering jaw. Now smile as wide as you
can and bring back teeth together. Still
smiling, lower and raise jaw 10 times
slowly. Relax and repeat once more. Feel
those muscles working.

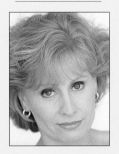

Body Beautiful

The skin on the rest of your body deserves attention, too. Don't forget:

Hands and nails Use hand cream all the time and always wear rubber gloves when you wash dishes or do housework. Prevent or minimize the brown age spots that sometimes appear on the backs of hands with either a retinol cream or with a hand mask made by mixing lemon juice with avocado. Keep nails attractive with a regular manicure. One marvelous benefit of hitting your middle years is your nails get stronger, so make the most of it.

Feet If you like to go barefoot, make sure you take care of your feet. They respond well to creams, massage, and exercise. The pain of hurting feet shows on your face, so if you must wear high heels, give your feet plenty of breaks by frequently changing into comfortable footwear.

Lips Keep lips well moisturized and protected against the sun with a UVA/B-rich balm or lipstick.

Teeth and gums Regular visits to the dental hygienist and dentist are a must; as are healthy food, plenty of vitamin C for healthy gums, scrupulous daily dental hygiene, and, if necessary, an approved whitening toothpaste for a bright smile.

Body skin Keep your body skin young by remembering it every now and then! Follow the routine here regularly and make sure to use gentle bath oils, gels, or creams in the bath or shower.

Relaxing essential oils

Bergamot, chamomile, clary, jasmine, lavender, neroli, sandalwood.

Invigorating essential oils

Basil, cinnamon, lemon, peppermint, pine, rosemary. (Essential oils are available from pharmacies and health food stores, and by mail order.)

20-Minute Skin Care Routine

1 Undress and put on your bathrobe. Cleanse face with gentle cleanser to suit skin type, using a cotton ball or a washcloth. (Photo A)

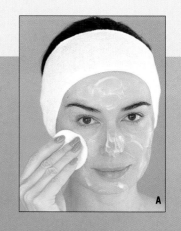

2 Steam face with head over bowl of steaming hot water for 2 minutes.

3 Apply moisturizing, purifying face mask. (Photo B).

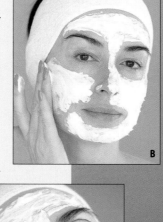

4 Bathe or shower with a few drops of relaxing essential oil or invigorating oil in the water. If you wish put used herbal tea bags, or cucumber or potato slices over your eyes. (Photo C). Relax totally for 10 minutes.

5 Pat body dry with thick warm towels. Apply body lotion all over while skin is still moist. Take special care of feet, knees, elbows, and neck.

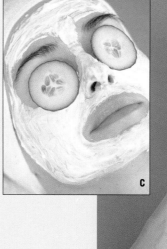

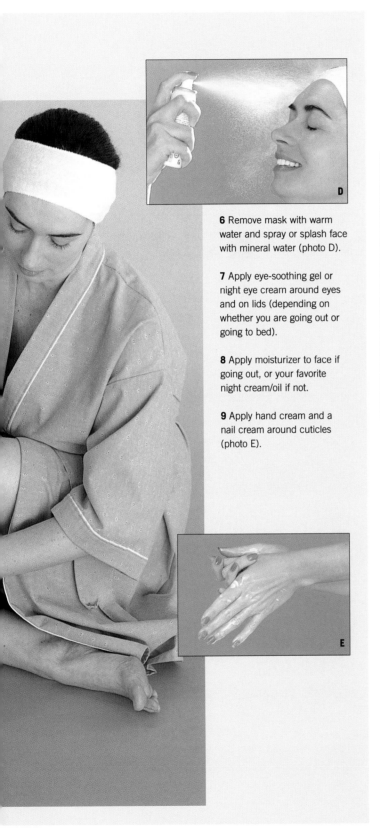

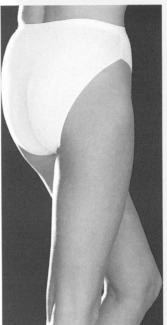

6 Remove mask with warm water and spray or splash face with mineral water (photo D).

7 Apply eye-soothing gel or night eye cream around eyes and on lids (depending on whether you are going out or going to bed).

8 Apply moisturizer to face if going out, or your favorite night cream/oil if not.

9 Apply hand cream and a nail cream around cuticles (photo E).

CELLULITE–WHAT WORKS?

Cellulite is the dimpled fat that appears on many women's lower bodies even if they aren't overweight. It isn't easy to get rid of but it can be done. Try these strategies and you will see a marked improvement in ten weeks–continue for further improvement.

• Do lower-body exercises–the most important single factor in cellulite control. Regular toning, aerobic, and stretch work for the legs (such as the routines within your 10-week program) are essential. The proof? Look at any woman who is at her correct weight and does plenty of lower-body work and you will rarely find cellulite.

• Maintain a correct body weight. Yes, it is true that thin women can get cellulite, but if you are overweight with cellulite, the cellulite won't go unless you get down to a reasonable weight.

• Eat healthily. I'm not a believer in the idea that cellulite is caused by toxins trapped in fat cells, but a diet such as the Zest Plan (page 103), rich in antioxidant vitamins and other vitamins and minerals and essential fatty acids, will help your skin maintain optimum condition.

• Massage cellulite regularly. Many tests have shown that if you massage cellulite using a rough mitt or loofah and a softening lotion or cream every day for a few weeks, the cellulite diminishes and the skin's appearance is improved. You have to massage regularly for several minutes at a time, and you have to do it firmly! There are many massage kits available, but you don't need to spend a lot. Just buy a loofah mitt and some ordinary body lotion–or dilute a little pure vitamin E oil in a base of almond oil . . . and start massaging.

*T*he right makeup can take years off. Conversely, the use of dated techniques, colors, and textures that are wrong for older skin can put years on. With the help of top makeup artist Celia Hunter, this workshop shows you how to make the most of your face.

WORKSHOP 6 # MAKEUP MAGIC

*C*elia says, "As you get older, you need to rethink your look every now and again. So many women stick with the same colors, brands, and types of cosmetics they have used throughout their adult life. But if you really look at your face, and look at the products now available, you may realize you are a long way from doing yourself justice with the products you use and the way you use them."

Even with the best skin-care routine, as described in Workshop 5, your skin and coloring change as you get older and the cosmetics that suit a 25-year-old will rarely suit a 45-year-old. Update your makeup with the following tips.

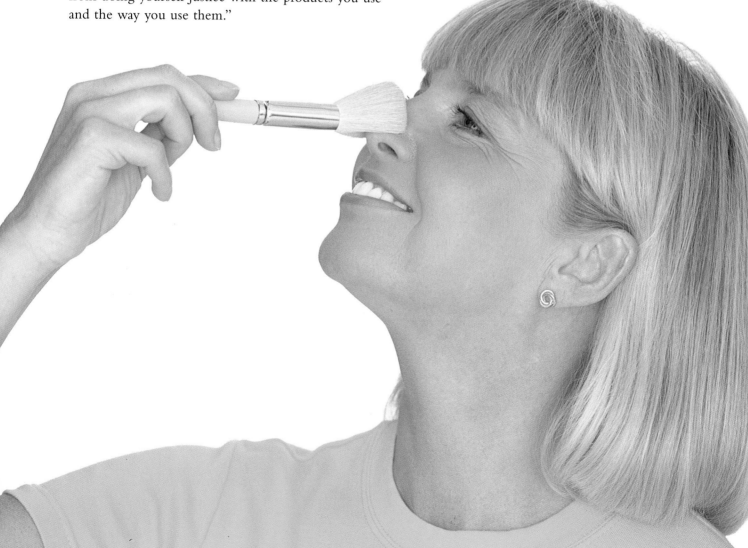

Updating Your Makeup

Heavy makeup

As your skin shows signs of aging—uneven patches of color, spider veins or dark circles, as well as fine lines—it is tempting to try a coverup job by piling on thicker foundation and more powder, or to focus attention on the eyes or lips by increasing the amount of shadow and liner or lipstick.

We've all seen the "whatever happened to Baby Jane?" syndrome on women of 45-plus, and it isn't a pretty sight. The truth is that a heavy hand when applying makeup isn't flattering at 35, let alone at 50 or 60. The general rule is "less is more," and the older you are, the lighter your touch should be. Particularly do not attempt to hide wrinkles as if you are filling cracks in a wall.

Luckily, help is at hand to disguise age-related face faults with minimum coverage (see "Catch Up with Makeup" on page 60).

Applying makeup in poor light

Few women have really decent light in which to apply makeup. And trying to do a good makeup job in the half-light of a gloomy bedroom in midwinter, for instance, is guaranteed to produce mistakes. Daylight will reveal brows badly penciled-in, blush applied too heavily, and so on. Invest in stage lights for your bathroom, or buy a makeup mirror with adjustable lighting. In summer, check your makeup by a window before going out the door.

Not taking your time

As we get older we need to pay more attention to the details of applying makeup, yet most women pay less. Sometimes I think it is because we have spent so many years making our faces up, that we're really a bit bored with the whole thing. We think we know our face so well, we can do in two minutes what used to take half an hour. And, of course, there are so many more important things to do than apply makeup, so we rush it. Don't. Blend foundation in very well; be scrupulous in dusting off any surplus powder; blend eyeshadow properly; apply thin coats of mascara rather than one thick coat in a glop; and pay special attention to applying lip color.

Think of your face now as a "new" face, and give it the attention you gave it when applying makeup for the very first time.

Using wrong colors

Skin changes tone as it ages, and so does hair. In general, they get paler. If you don't adjust your makeup colors to match this change, you'll look harsh and/or drained. For example, I used to wear dark brown eyeshadow to diminish my slightly protruding eyes and create a socket where none existed. For interest, I tried a similar shade on my eyes the other day—and looked just awful, as if I'd been in a fight and lost.

Dark colors are drab on most older faces, and black, in particular, is a no-no unless you are very dark-complexioned. Throw out your black mascara and black eyeliner; it is no longer what you need.

Vivid colors, too, can be unflattering, hard, and draining. You may, for example, be olive-complexioned with dark hair and have always enjoyed wearing fire-engine red lipstick. Try a softer red with a hint of pink or blue or brown in it—I bet it will suit you better. Blondes, also, often wear red lipstick, but it's rarely the best option for someone over 40. Flattering makeup for your face should enhance, not dominate! Ideal colors are neutrals or neutral bases with a blended color in light to medium tones. For more on you and color, turn to Workshop 9.

Using shimmer and shine

As a general rule, the older you are, the more important it is to avoid shimmer, shine, frost, and gloss on your face. Shimmer and frost just draw attention to wrinkles, bags, and crepey skin. The worst mistake of all is frosted eye shadow on your lids if there is any hint of crepiness in them.

Throw out all such things from your makeup shelf and go for silky mattes for your eyes, lips, and face. The new high-tech cosmetics (see "Catch Up with Makeup," overleaf) provide exactly the right textures and colors for you, so why not use them?

Old techniques

If you are still shading in the same socket lines you did 20 years ago and have never parted with your painted-on eyelashes or black liner inside your lower lids, you're stuck in a time warp! Use the information in this workshop (and in women's magazines) to update your techniques. You should also avoid using blusher to shape your face; using a foundation several shades darker than your skin tone to mimic a tan or add color; using a dark lip liner and filling in the center in a pale color; and other unfortunate makeup tricks. At 16 you can almost get away with it but, at 45, never.

Changing the way you look at your face
Because you see your face every day, and because the changes happen so gradually, you may not notice them. So if you are still using the same techniques you did ages ago, you need to sit in front of a good mirror and make an honest appraisal of yourself. This should include the shape of your face (pull your hair back and if you're not sure, draw an outline on the mirror in lipstick around your face); the condition and tone of your skin (to help you decide on the right color foundation and powder); your eye type (large, small, deep set, wide apart, etc.); the under-eye area (do you have any dark circles, bags, deep wrinkles?); your lips (plump and smooth or thin and wrinkled; balanced top and bottom or unbalanced?), and so on. Write down all your good points and those you consider less than ideal. With the right makeup you can enhance the good points and play down the imperfect ones. You'll discover specific makeup tricks to correct those less-than-perfect features in the following pages.

Best of all, take a trip to the cosmetic department and spend as much time as you can checking out all the cosmetics on display. Try out colors and see what you like and dislike; what suits and what doesn't. Try foundations for maximum coverage with minimum depth. Try everything you can. It really is the best way to update your look. Take advantage of the free makeovers that many cosmetics companies offer. Some are better than others, but you will certainly learn a lot. Whether you've always worn makeup or never have before, it's a good way to experiment with new products for a new look.

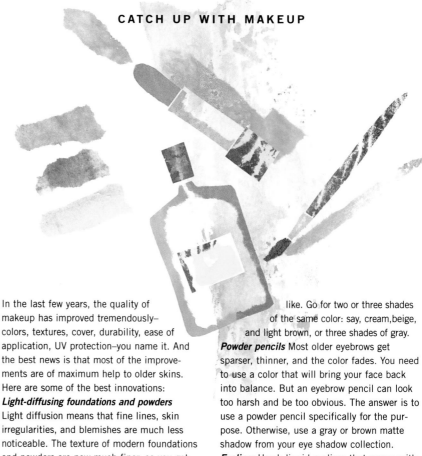

CATCH UP WITH MAKEUP

In the last few years, the quality of makeup has improved tremendously–colors, textures, cover, durability, ease of application, UV protection–you name it. And the best news is that most of the improvements are of maximum help to older skins. Here are some of the best innovations:

Light-diffusing foundations and powders
Light diffusion means that fine lines, skin irregularities, and blemishes are much less noticeable. The texture of modern foundations and powders are now much finer, so you get greater coverage while using less–terrific for older skins. Many foundations now offer UVA and UVB protection and other pluses, such as antioxidants, alpha-hydroxy acids (AHA) and moisturizers.

Concealers A decade or so ago, my concealer was a solid, rock-hard stick that came in two shades, very light or dark, dragged on the skin, and was probably more of an eyesore than the odd blemish or dark circles under the eyes I was trying to hide. The new concealers are great, especially the liquid ones you apply with a finger or a small applicator.

Corn silk powder If you have coarse skin or an oily T-zone, corn silk powder is wonderful. It is so fine, it gives great coverage without clogging.

Pick-your-own eye shadow palettes Various cosmetic companies offer the empty shadow cases that you fill with two, three, or more, colors of your choice, thus banishing the need to buy a lot of colors just to get the one you like. Go for two or three shades of the same color: say, cream, beige, and light brown, or three shades of gray.

Powder pencils Most older eyebrows get sparser, thinner, and the color fades. You need to use a color that will bring your face back into balance. But an eyebrow pencil can look too harsh and be too obvious. The answer is to use a powder pencil specifically for the purpose. Otherwise, use a gray or brown matte shadow from your eye shadow collection.

Eyeliner Harsh liquid eyeliner that comes with a thick brush and dries the second you've applied it (too thickly, of course!) is not for anyone over 35. If your eyes need a little gentle outlining, buy an eyeliner in a soft brown or gray shade. Some can be blended in before they dry to soften the line.

Lip pencils With age you tend to get fine lines around your lips into which lipstick can "bleed" through the day and which, quite frankly, looks awful. To avoid this use a lip pencil in a natural shade and fill in (for more on this see the makeovers that follow). There are also numerous lip foundations that prevent lipstick bleed.

Lip colorings As someone who hates the "wet mouth" syndrome, I love the new lip colors that add color without feeling slick. These suit most older complexions very well. A lip pencil will do the same trick if you use it all over rather than just to outline, but may not last as long as a lip color.

THE 30S

Makeover for Sue

1 Sue's skin didn't need heavy foundation—just a little tinted moisturizer to match her natural skin color, gently blended well with fingers or a damp sponge.
2 A touch of concealer around the eyes and nose hid her few dark shadows.
3 Celia applied very fine loose powder all over with a big brush, then brushed off any surplus.
4 Eye shadow was kept simple—a rust-brown powder applied on the lash line, then blended up and out slightly to give the "hardly there" look.
5 Two thin coats of dark brown mascara finished the eyes.
6 Celia used a touch of pink-beige blush on the cheekbones to bring out their natural structure and to help Sue's eyes sparkle.
7 To finish, a creamy rose-pink lipstick—no need for lip liner as Sue does not have any fine lines around her lips.

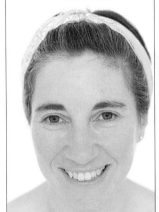

BEFORE: Sue with no makeup on.

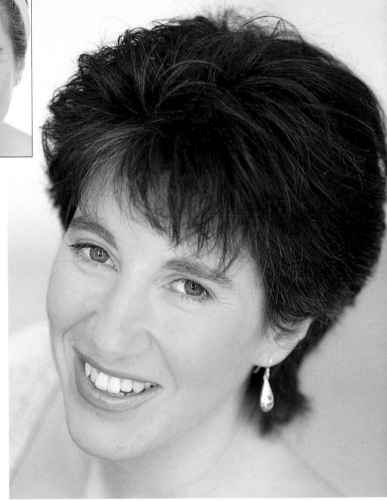

AFTER
With brows plucked (Celia just thinned them by taking out a few hairs all over) and lips colored to draw more attention to her neat, slim jawline, Sue's face has really come alive.

Says Celia:
"This is a simple, seven-step makeup that anyone can do in five minutes or so at home."

Says Sue:
"I feel like a completely new person. Isn't it amazing what makeup can do!"

Thirty-nine-year-old Sue normally doesn't wear any makeup at all. "I have never worn it, and don't have any confidence in applying it, either." Celia promised a natural look that Sue could easily copy. **Celia's analysis:** "Sue has a strong, good face with high cheekbones and a nice oval shape. Without makeup, her brows tend to dominate her features and hide her very attractive eyes, which can look green, blue, or gray, depending on the light. Her nose is good, maybe slightly long, and her mouth is well-shaped, too, but with a slightly short top lip.

"Sue's skin is neither oily nor dry, and with a healthy even tone and few blemishes. For many women, their 30s can be their skin's best years, especially if they suffered from oily skin in their teens and 20s. As long as they moisturize regularly, there may be little sign of wrinkles. Makeup should be slightly more subtle than in the 20s, but skin tone has yet to fade, and so changes can be minimal."

THE 40S

Hilary's new look

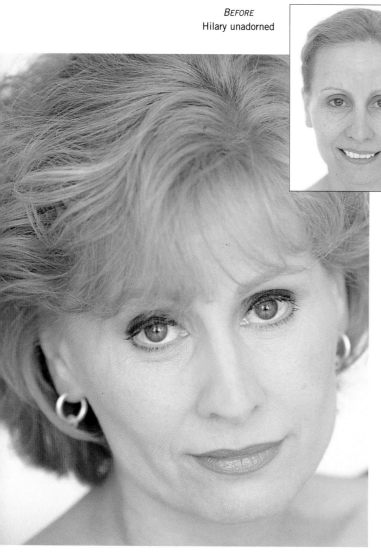

BEFORE
Hilary unadorned

Hilary, 43, has always enjoyed wearing makeup; but now, heading into her mid-40s, she needs to reconsider her penchant for dark eye shadows. However, she is skeptical that lighter colors will do anything for her face.

Celia's analysis: "Hilary has a very good face–square but well balanced, with fabulous cheekbones and strong features. Her eyes are lovely–big, blue, and expressive, but there's quite a lot of shadowing and darkness around them which can be easily rectified. Her skin and lips can be quite dry without regular deep moisturizing, so I'm going to get as much moisture into her makeup as I can.

"Hilary's skin is typical of her age for someone with fair hair. There are some fine lines around the eyes (which the darker colors tend to accentuate) and the mouth, but no deep wrinkles. She has a few spider veins here and there but not much to worry about. Her skin is sensitive, so I'm going to use hypoallergenic cosmetics and apply them very gently.

"Be sure to wash your applicators, powder puffs, sponges, and so on regularly. Makeup, dirt, and grease can build up on them and cause problems, especially if you have sensitive skin."

1 Celia applied a hydrating liquid foundation with medium coverage all over Hilary's face, including the eyelids and brow bone, but used slightly less around the eyes and mouth to avoid any trace of heaviness there.
2 Concealer was applied to the inner eyes and the undereye dark circles and on any spider veins. Always use concealer after foundation and before powder.
3 Next, a minimum dusting of ultrafine loose powder, just to take any shine off, especially down the nose and on the forehead.
4 Celia created a soft eye-liner effect by using a charcoal gray powder eye shadow applied along the upper lash line with a small wet brush and blended to soften.
5 Hilary has a good natural eye socket which Celia enhanced with a soft red-brown powder shadow, blended above and below to soften.
6 Charcoal powder shadow was applied lightly under the lower lashes.
7 Celia used brown-black mascara, with a light hand. "Avoid lash-building mascaras which can clump; a look you really don't want."
8 A warm terracotta blush on the cheekbones lifts Hilary's fair skin and gives her a healthy glow.
9 Lips were outlined with a nearly nude lip pencil and then filled in with a pale pink with a hint of peach, then blotted with a tissue to give a more natural finish.

AFTER
A glamorous, yet soft, look to her makeup has brought out Hilary's natural beauty.

Says Celia:
"Fair-haired, light-eyed women–especially those over 40–very rarely look good in dark browns and black. As I thought, a lighter touch has enhanced Hilary's looks, rather than detract from them."

Says Hilary:
"I'd been using the same makeup colors for years. I'm so glad Celia has shown me they were no longer right."

THE 50S

Glamour for Pam

As they get older, many women try to disguise skin faults and paleness by ladling on more makeup than ever before, which is just what you shouldn't do. Thick foundation imbeds itself in wrinkles and makes them seem more pronounced. But you can still look both glamorous and beautiful, as Pam, at 57, shows. **Celia's analysis:** "Pamela has good skin for her age, a little dry with a few broken capillaries, but fine skin quality.

Around and after menopause, skin texture can change, becoming coarser, with enlarged pores and more dry patches. Wrinkles tend to deepen, too. For enlarged pores, I recommend regular use of a face mask especially for this skin type, but on the enlarged-pore areas only. A mild scrub specially formulated for dry skin is also good. For dry and/or wrinkled areas, obviously moisturize properly every day and night, and use hydrating cosmetics.

"The best way to apply makeup to wrinkles is to put as little on them as possible. Begin blending foundation onto your nose and midface area, then smooth it to the outer parts of the face so they receive lighter coverage.

"By their 50s most women will need to tone their colors down again. Pam's face is a rounded heart shape, and all her features are soft, dainty, delicate. Her current makeup is a bit tired and dowdy. She needs more modern colors and products to bring her up to date and add a little drama to her softness."

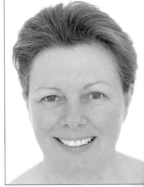

BEFORE
Pam before her makeup session

1 Celia used a medium-coverage foundation slightly warmer than Pam's natural skin-tone, applying hardly any to her outer eye area.
2 The foundation was dusted with very fine loose powder and the surplus powder brushed off.
3 Celia applied a medium brown powder eye shadow to the socket and corner of Pam's eyes to give her heavy lids a lift.
4 A soft coral-pink shadow followed, blended in below the brows and in the center of the lid to give sparkle.
5 A little medium-gray eye pencil was used to give definition under the outer edge of the lower lashes.
6 Dark brown mascara, lightly applied to upper and lower lashes, opens up the eyes.
7 Warm pink-toned powder blush gives a hint of color to Pam's cheeks.
8 Celia outlined Pam's lips with a lip pencil one shade darker than her natural lip color, then filled in with a coral cream lipstick and blotted with tissue to finish.

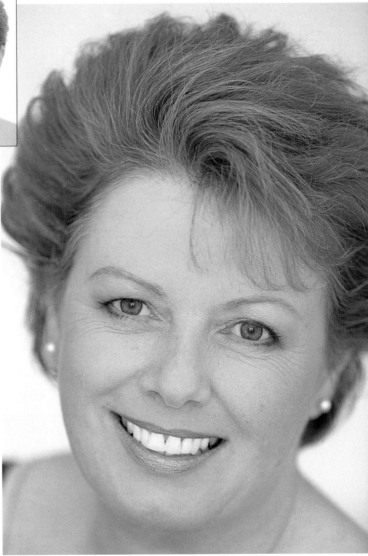

AFTER
Says Celia:
"Well, I have to say, Pam is gorgeous! This shows how small changes can make a big difference."

Says Pam:
"Yes, I do like it. It's more makeup than I'd normally wear, and yet it feels and looks light."

Face Furniture

More women over 40 wear glasses (at least some of the time) than don't. Yet we pay little attention to them. The right glasses should enhance your looks, not send you into a tailspin every time you put them on.

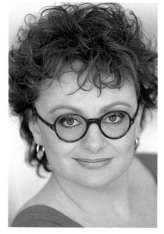

Sal Houston, above, has worn glasses for years and had chosen her heavy, dark-rimmed, round specs to go with her dark hair–but they weren't doing her any favors. Says stylist Ceril Campbell, "Sal doesn't need a disguise, which is what these glasses are. They are overpowering and hiding her face." Below, Sal tries on some glasses to see which suit her and which are mistakes.

Here's the perfect pair of specs for Sal; they suit her, and her new hairstyle. Now we can see what you look like, Sally!

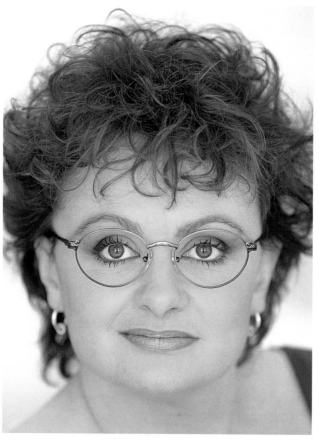

Tips:

● *Buy new frames as often as you can. Think of glasses as a fashion accessory (but don't fall for wildly eccentric ones–not everyone may get the joke).*

● *Take into consideration your hairstyle and face shape. Small hair, small face–small glasses! Big hair, big face–big glasses!*

● *Consider your coloring–eyes, skin, hair. Few fair people can wear heavy, dark frames.*

● *Don't choose frames in a color that doesn't go with most of your clothes (unless you're buying several pairs). For example, why buy blue frames if you never wear blue?*

● *Remember your jewelery. If you like to wear silver near your face, don't choose gold frames, and vice versa.*

● *Try on lots of frames before deciding–you'll soon realize which frame shapes suit your face.*

● *Consider contact lenses. Although everyone can look great in the right glasses, contact lenses can be a real confidence booster.*

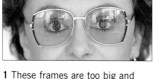

1 These frames are too big and angular for Sal's small face. Her own glasses are a better shape and a rounder frame will soften her squarish jaw-line. Let's try some lighter, oval frames . . .

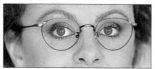

2 These green frames suit Sal well. If you wear glasses all the time, you should consider having more than one pair and changing them to match your outfit or the occasion. If you can't afford to do that, though, stick to a neutral color that suits you well.

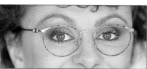

3 These glasses don't suit Sal's face–the tops of the frames should always echo the line of the brow–slightly above it is all right, but never below it.

Quick Tricks for Younger Looks

Makeup, as well as all the things you learned in Workshop 5, can help minimize the subtle changes your face undergoes as it ages.

Heavy jaw Faces tend to "slip" a bit, as the years pass, making the jawline heavier than it used to be. Camouflage this by wearing eye makeup (not too dark) and blush to direct attention to the upper part of your face. For evening, you can shade under the chin and along the jawline with a slightly darker foundation. But do this carefully and don't try it during the daytime.

Small or tired eyes As we get older, lids tend to sag, causing the eyes to look smaller. Frequently you can look tired even when you are not. Help to correct this by choosing a white or cream-colored soft eye pencil and dot the color at the inside corner of each eye, over foundation and before powdering, and blending well. Also dot the pencil between upper and lower lashes at the outer corners. If using eyeliner, never extend it so the upper and lower lines join at this outer edge. Always leave this gap and fill in with the light pencil. Use color on your lids and use blush on your cheeks, which always brightens up the eyes.

Thin lips Aging causes thinning of the lips. If this doesn't suit you, you can make them look fuller by taking a lip pencil in a shade barely darker than your own lip color and outlining the lips just outside (but only just outside) the natural lip line. Fill in with more lip pencil, then a touch of creamy lipstick. If one lip is thinner than the other, use the same trick but on the thin lip only. You could also use a slightly darker shade on the thicker lip, as dark colors diminish.

Lip bleed Stop lipstick from sliding into the fine lines around your mouth by using a lip pencil or a lip tint rather than a creamy or glossy lipstick. If using lipstick, use a long-lasting formula and always blot after applying. Or try one of the new lip foundations under your lip color.

Pale, tired complexion If exercise, fresh air, and sleep don't work, add color to your face with a tiny amount of tanning cream and/or a dusting of blush on the top of the cheeks. Eye and lip shades (and clothes) that flatter your coloring will give you a real lift (see "Color Confidence" on page 78).

Tricks not to try . . .

Some things are best left alone . . .

Celia says, "Even for the camera, I never try to correct face shapes by shading. It is so easy for everyone else to see what you've been trying to do that it draws more attention to the "problem." Unless you are a professional, it is very hard to achieve a natural result. That's why I won't do it on my makeovers–I don't like to do anything that a woman can't copy at home."

The best solution to problems such as saggy eyelids, eye bags, nose-to-mouth line, and poor chin definition is facial exercises (see page 55). Done daily they do bring results.

TOP 10 WAYS TO TAKE YEARS OFF YOUR FACE INSTANTLY

1. Use blush.
2. Get enough sleep and exercise.
3. Pluck and use brow color on your eyebrows.
4. Wear a pair of flattering earrings.
5. Wear less foundation and powder.
6. Pick a flattering hairstyle (see Workshop 7).
7. Just occasionally put eye drops of Murine or similar in your eyes.
8. Wear makeup colors that suit your skin, hair, and eye coloring (see Workshop 9).
9. Make sure your glasses are up to date and flattering.
10. Smile.

*F*or this workshop, I've enlisted the help of leading hairdresser Paul Edmonds. Paul, who cut and styled all our models' hair and provided much of the advice that appears in this workshop, appears regularly on TV style shows; he styles for movies and counts top models, actors, and TV personalities among his many famous clients. He has his own line of aromatherapy hair products. Paul has the most common-sense approach to hair I have found in any hairdresser. He has an unfailing instinct for knowing what style will suit a woman and her hair type, and also recognizes that most of us can't afford the time or money to spend hours on our hair. So read on with confidence, and get the inspiration you need.

WORKSHOP 7 — HAIR FLAIR 1—SUPERSTYLES

Four Top Hair Swaps to Take off Years

*W*hether you want your hair long, medium, or short, straight or curly, there's a right and a wrong way to wear it! In our "before" and "after" photos the difference is sometimes very small–but the result is wonderful.

GOOD-BYE TO CURTAINS

*K*ay is 49 but still wants to wear her hair long. No problem. Says Paul, "You can wear your hair long at almost any age, as long as it is in good condition and well-styled. But be careful to avoid the curtain effect of straight sides (see below left) which drag the face down, and the flat-top caused by the sheer weight of long hair."

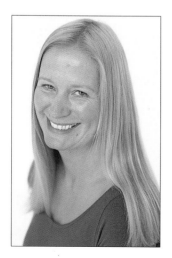

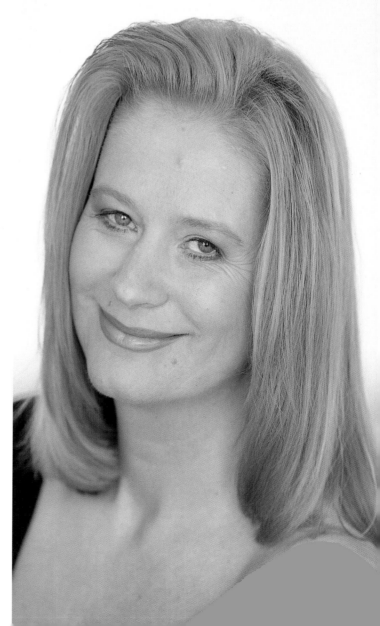

SWAP: Paul has taken a few inches off Kay's hair and graduated the sides. Before drying, he applied volumizer for fine, limp hair and then had Kay bend forward so he could blow-dry to give the hair lift. "Kay is narrow at the temple, with a wide jaw, so we need to finish the style by lifting the hair at the temple and slightly turning the graduated ends into the face."

The result–a stunning transformation which Kay loves and will have no problem re-creating at home. All she needs is a trim every eight weeks.

TAKING IT UP

Change your look in a minute! For an instant facelift, sweep long hair on top of your head. Angela, 40, has very thick hair that she wants to leave long. However, the curtain effect and hard forehead line are accentuating her oblong face and not doing her any favors. When you think of youthful flattering hair, think of height and light.

LENGTH WITH LIFT

A medium-to-long layered look is good for most faces and a good compromise between long hair and short. But most women tend to wear this style too long, producing a flat top and bushy sides that don't flatter. Linda, 47, has a very attractive face but her nice eyes and bone structure are being diminished by too much shapeless hair. "I tend to use heated rollers every day, otherwise it looks a mess," she says. Paul says, "The top doesn't gel with the bottom; the hair is a bit too long at the sides for Linda's face, and it's too curly and slightly old-fashioned. Heated rollers tend to give this effect unless you are very careful."

SWAP: Paul trimmed, conditioned, and colored Angela's hair (see page 72) but agreed she would look terrific with it upswept. The quickest and easiest way to put hair up is to bend forward, brush all the hair forward, grab it on the crown, and put it through a scrunchie. Leave the ends loose or twist them around and secure with pins. Pull some strands of hair out around your hairline to soften the effect and you have a look that you can wear anywhere.

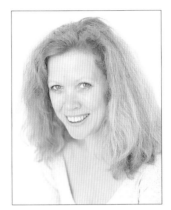

SWAP: Paul took the length off the sides and cut the top and bangs to give a more flattering, less heavy look to Linda's hair. From the back, however, the length appears to be exactly the same as before. Paul blow-dried using a round brush to create a soft, wispy, feathered look. Linda is going to try this at home and banish those heated rollers.

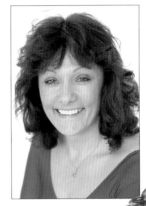

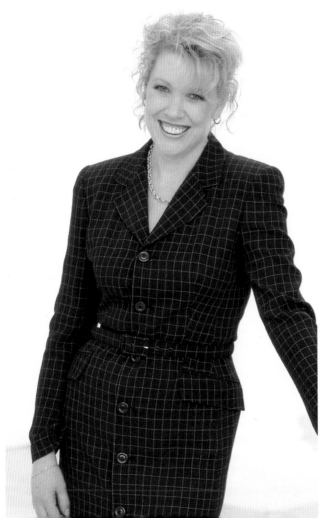

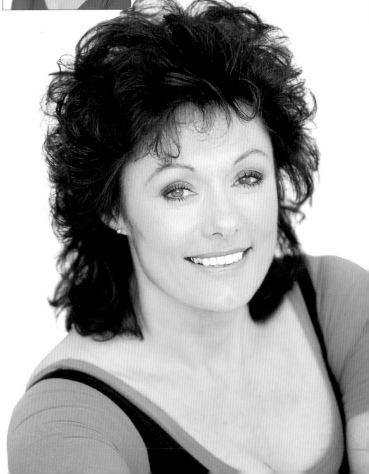

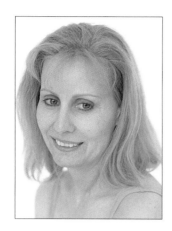

GOING FOR THE CHOP

Hilary, 43, has very nice fair hair which she's been wearing in a shoulder-length bob for years. Paul says, "This style is rather limp and heavy, and manages to make Hilary's lovely face rather unnoticeable. We want a definite style that will complement her strong features. We need to focus the impact on her eyes and cheekbones.

"It's a brave woman who will go for a short style after years of having it long or mid length, but I'm going to leave plenty of length through Hilary's hair on top so it won't be that much of a shock! She has very full, naturally curly hair that will hold the style very well if I shorten the length around the sides and blend it in to the longer hair on top."

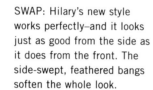

SWAP: Hilary's new style works perfectly–and it looks just as good from the side as it does from the front. The side-swept, feathered bangs soften the whole look.

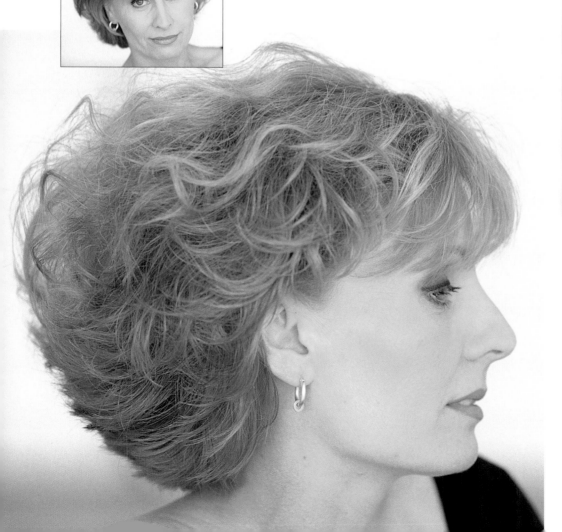

THE INSTANT FACELIFT HAIR CODE

• Don't keep too much length below the jawline.

• Think "light and height"– go for feathered layers and more hair on top of the head than below the chin.

• Avoid the "curtains" effect.

• Avoid flatness on the crown – think lift and "body."

• Don't pull hair back severely from the face–keep it quite soft.

• Light and layered bangs almost always look better than blunt, heavy bangs.

• Think uplift – hair brushed upwards is always more flattering than hair drooping down.

• Lighten the color around the face (*see Workshop 8*).

New Looks for Old
– A potpourri of ideas to help you make the most of your hair

Things to be wary of . . .

● Perms. Bubble hairstyles are unflattering and a real age giveaway. If you really do need a perm to give body to fine, thin hair, make sure it is a soft one and that the hairdresser avoids the bubble effect at all cost. Pamela's hair had been frequently permed after being cut quite short and consequently you could see her scalp at the crown where the hair fell away into sections. We persuaded her to grow it out (see page 71) and then, with Paul's clever cutting and straight styling, it looked much more up-to-date.

● The "set" look. Don't let any hairdresser set your hairstyle into a rock-hard helmet. Up-to-date hair needs to have movement.

● The same style if you've had it more than five years. Paul says, "People like to stay within their own comfort zone, and this often means sticking with the same old style. Often, just a very slight change in the way your hair is cut and/or styled can update it. Time-warp hair is very aging. Women tend to keep up with hair trends in their teens and 20s, then at 30-plus, stick with the same old thing. If your style can be dated by other people, then so can you! "Also, your style may no longer suit you. Take a good long look at your face and ask yourself if you couldn't do better. Few people can wear just one style throughout their lives."

● Keeping hair long at all costs. Long hair can suit older women, but it needs to be thick and glossy and sleek and cared for very well. Long scruffy, scraggly hair on a woman of 40 or 50 will have people sniggering, not admiring.

Choosing a new style

1 Use Paul's guidelines on the previous three pages.

2 Look at magazines, catalogs, and newspapers, and cut out styles you like to take to the hairdresser for reference.

3 Look at other women's hair and if you see someone with a style you love, ask her where she got it cut and get the name of the stylist. Go there.

4 Talk with the hairdresser; tell him or her what look you'd like and show photos if you can. Be prepared for the hairdresser to adapt this look, or perhaps even tell you it won't suit your hair type. For example, Kay's hair (on pages 66 and opposite) would never cut and style like Hilary's hair; it is far too fine and soft.

5 Remember, you've got to style your hair at home, so don't go for anything you will find difficult to duplicate or care for.

6 Discuss your face and body shape with your hairdresser and try to choose a style that will suit both. If your face is long and thin, go for a short style with width at the sides, for example. A round face (see Pamela's "after" photo, page 71) looks best with short hair given body on top. A square or oblong face needs softening with hair wisps around the face and curved (perhaps flicked up) lines, softly layered–even an inch or two of layering cut into the bottom may be enough.

7 Your head shape is also important. A style with body can disguise a flat head, for example. Wash your hair and use two mirrors to view your head from all angles.

S o you've got the right style – but what kind of condition is your hair in? Could it benefit from a color change or enhancement? If you're going gray, what is the best course of action? In this workshop, with the help of Paul and his colorist Tracey, we find the answers.

WORKSHOP
8 HAIR FLAIR 2
COLOR AND CONDITION

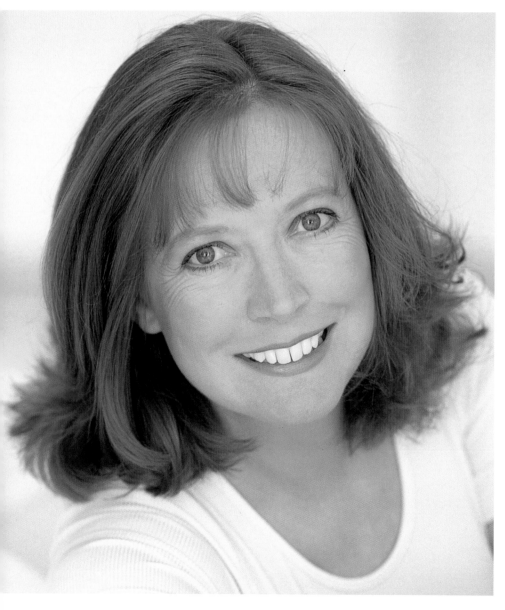

Natural color that's faded:

Don't feel you are selling out if you decide to get your hair colored after years of leaving it natural. It's really no more of a "cheat" than wearing makeup or having your teeth fixed. After years of being fortunate enough to have a thick head of natural chestnut hair, I took the plunge for the first time recently when I realized I was no longer chestnut but more of a nondescript brown. It took me two seconds to get over the shock of the new color and now I'm really pleased (see left).

Don't worry that your hair may turn a nasty shade of bright orange. Go to a reputable colorist–personal recommendation is the best course. If anything is slightly wrong, or if you dislike the results, speak up! It can usually be easily corrected. If you opt for a semi-permanent color at first, as opposed to a permanent color, it will wash out after about 10 washes.

Most women whose hair color has naturally faded will want to return to their original color. If you were dark-haired, you could take this opportunity to choose a slightly lighter shade. Very dark hair can be too harsh on a mature woman. As you get older, your skin color changes, your makeup should be softer, and so should your hair.

TIME FOR A COLOR CHANGE?

Your hair and appearance may benefit from a change of color if you fit into any of the following categories:

- Natural color that's faded.
- You've been coloring your hair for ages but wonder if the color still suits you.
- Dull hair or a general feeling that you need brightening up.
- Various degrees of gray.

You've been coloring your hair for ages:

As you get older, a good hair color, like a good hair style, is one that has the effect of "lighting" your face. Colors that aren't always ideal, then, are one-dimensional, too dark, or too harsh. What suited you five years ago may not suit you now.

Pamela had been having a single tone golden blonde permanent color on her hair for years, which looked solid and lacked lightness.

"My natural color was mousy, but I expect I am quite gray now; not that I'd know, as I haven't seen my real hair color in ages!" she said.

Paul and Tracey explained that a much more flattering effect would be achieved by using three different colors all through her hair in complementing shades. Pam was dubious–"I don't want to end up like a tabby cat!" she said.

Little over an hour later, she was delighted. Tracey had used a rich gold, a light gold, and a dark gold applied in streaks of color. The finished effect is very natural and quite stunning.

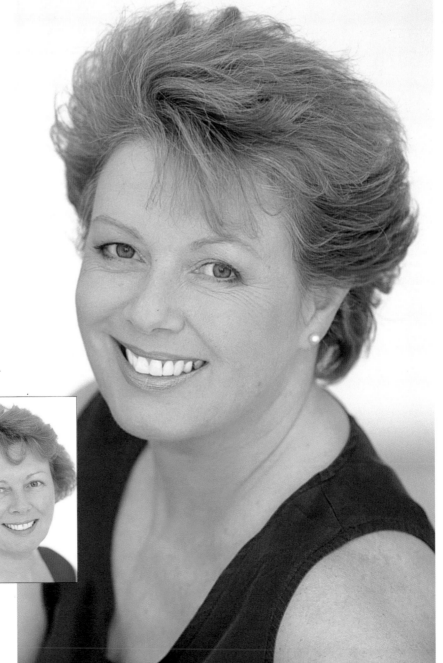

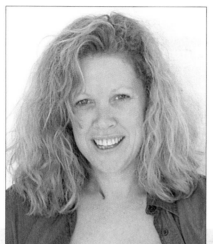

Angela had dull, blonde, thick-textured hair, which needed both deep conditioning and lightening. Tracey bleached thick sections of the hair around the front and top, and a few underneath, so Angela can put her hair up, then added a soft blonde tint. Afterward, she used an intensive conditioner to smooth the hair cuticles and add gloss.

Dull hair or a general feeling that you need brightening up:

Dull hair can be partly rectified by proper conditioning (see page 75) but it can also be changed with color. The tips we gave for correcting faded hair apply here as well, but you can also consider adding just a hint of color with vegetable dyes, which wash out in a few washes, or the shampoo-in temporary colorants you can do yourself. These will add shine and a hint of color which washes out in two or three shampoos (unless you use them every shampoo, in which case the color builds up).

You should also consider low-lights, adding deep colors in streaks; highlights, which Tracey did for Angela, or "tips," which she did for Sal. Highlights added to dark blonde to medium brown or mousy hair can be very effective, producing a light and bright look that takes off years from your appearance.

Sal's hair carried a permanent reddish-brown tint that looked lifeless. Tracey decided to brighten the hair around the face by tipping. She bleached just the tips of the hair and then added an auburn vegetable dye over all the hair, including the bleached tips. The result is a glossier, redder color on most of the hair, but paler at the ends.

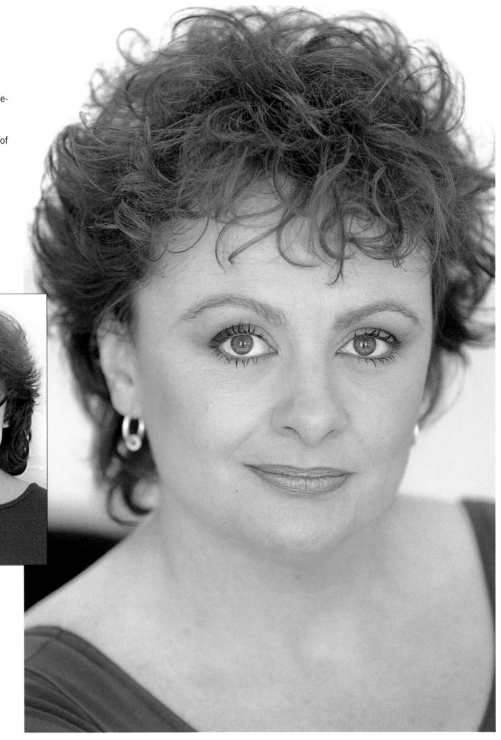

Various degrees
of gray:

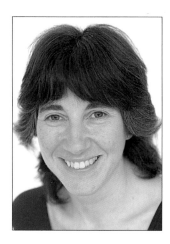

Gray hair suits some women and if you are one of those, it is fine to leave it–but only if you take care to keep it in tip-top condition because, as Paul points out, gray hair is often dull and without any shine.

"Gray hair isn't actually gray at all," says Paul. "It is white. But because it is mixed with the darker hair that still contains pigment, it looks gray. One reason gray hair can look attractive is because the color suits the paler tones of mature skin.

"However, I'd say that 80 percent of the time, it is best to color it. But I would very rarely do a solid color on its own. I'd add color and then highlights afterward, which can be very subtle. If someone has gone gray, I would also use a light-to-warm color–not a dark one."

Most women who notice the first signs of gray appearing in their otherwise nicely colored hair during their 30s and 40s, tend to leave it alone, or cover it with a semi-permanent color to match their own color. But, the more gray that appears, the less successful this will be.

Sue (left) is 39 and had quite a lot of gray hair at the sides but virtually none on top or at the back. Even after cutting, her side panels of gray were still apparent. She wanted to be rid of them but didn't want a permanent color all over her nearly-black hair. The answer was simple–Tracey used a semipermanent color, in dark brown, on those side panels and left the rest alone. She did use a reddish wash-out vegetable dye on all the hair to add gloss. Sue was extremely pleased with the result.

If you have a lot of gray hair and want a change but nothing drastic, choose a light color or, preferably, two or three colors mixed as Tracey did for Pamela (page 71).

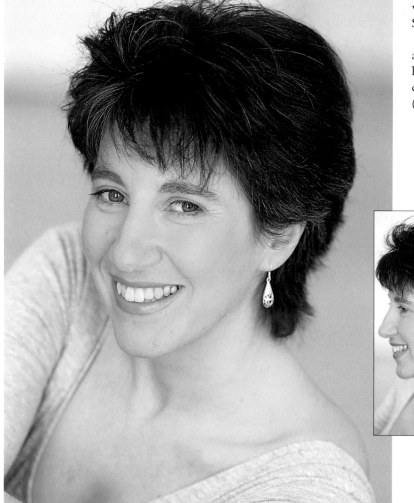

CONDITION UPDATE

Whatever your age and the current state of your hair, it shouldn't be difficult to get it in good condition and keep it that way. Here are the solutions to the most frequently asked hair condition questions.

Q My hair is oily at the scalp and dry at the ends. Is there a conditioner to deal with both problems at once?

A There are some that claim to condition only where it is needed, but in my experience the best solution is to simply condition the ends of the hair and leave the roots alone. Also, get trimmed regularly to cut off those dry ends.

Q Is there such a thing as product build-up on hair. If so, what should I do about it?

A If you use a lot of leave-in conditioners, and styling products, there will be buildup on the hair. When you wash your hair, they will be removed. Some shampoos claim specifically to remove buildup, but any shampoo should do the trick.

Q Can your hair get used to certain shampoos or other products so they work less effectively after a time?

A Some experts say yes, others say no. The simple solution is if your usual products are working well, continue with them. But if your hair is being difficult, dry, over-oily, frizzy, or whatever, for no reason you can think of, by all means try something new (trial-size first). Hair does change and you can't expect to go on using the same products forever with the same results.

Q Can my diet affect my hair condition?

A Yes. A healthy diet like the Zest Plan (page 103) will give hair its best chance of being healthy, too. You need enough protein, vitamins, minerals, and essential fatty acids in your diet. Many women report better hair condition when they have been taking evening primrose or starflower oil for a while. Poor diet can lead to dull, dry, brittle hair.

Q Can heat affect hair condition?

A Yes. Electrical hair tools, if used too often and at too high a temperature, too close to the hair, will dry it out and cause split ends. The answer is to use them with caution. Keep the hairdryer at least 8 inches away from your hair and use blow-dry lotion or leave-in conditioner. Use heated rollers only occasionally and consider buying some of the new ones with a low-heat setting.

Q My hair's been in poor condition since I began swimming regularly. What can I do?

A Chlorine will strip moisture from your hair, as will the sea, bleach, and even the sun. You can buy a preswim conditioner, which you apply to your hair thickly and which forms a barrier while you swim. (I agree that swimming caps are not the most elegant or comfortable of things.) In fact, any thick cream conditioner will do this job, although if you're in the water long enough, eventually it will wear off. After swimming, rinse and wash hair immediately and use an intensive conditioner. You can buy brands especially formulated to counteract the effect of chlorine. A weekly deep conditioning treatment (wrap your hair in a hot towel to help it work) is also a good idea.

Q Any solution for making frizzy hair look sleek?

A After shampooing, condition it thoroughly, then rinse and use an antifrizz styling lotion. While blow-drying with a heated styling brush on LOW, use your free hand to keep smoothing the hair down as you dry. Also try a silicone-based hair serum–a little of this nongreasy lotion goes a long way.

Q My hair has become more coarse over the last year or two. I am 48. Why is this?

A Hair does tend to become coarser in some women. Others find it thins and becomes finer. Hormonal changes around menopause are the most likely answer. For coarse hair the only thing you can do is make sure to keep it very well conditioned to keep it supple and give it shine. Fine, thinning, limp, or shapeless hair will benefit from correct cutting (short hair generally looks best), and the use of volumizers or mousse when styling.

Q Which is the best moisturizer for dry hair?

A Almost impossible to answer. But certainly, you don't have to spend a fortune. Like face creams, it is more important to use a conditioner regularly, use enough to cover all your hair (unless you're not conditioning the roots), and follow the instructions. Conditioner also works best in a warm atmosphere. Try various trial-size or packet conditioners until you find one that suits your hair. Or, if your hair condition is fabulous after you've been to the hairdresser, you could purchase the products they use, which are usually available to buy.

C eril Campbell is a top style adviser. She makes over TV news anchors, has her own style slot on Sky TV, and has helped countless TV viewers and magazine readers to find their own best looks. Ceril had great fun persuading our 10-week participants to rethink their clothes for Workshops 9 and 10. The results speak for themselves…

WORKSHOP *9*

STYLE ASSESSMENT 1
FINDING YOUR OWN STYLE

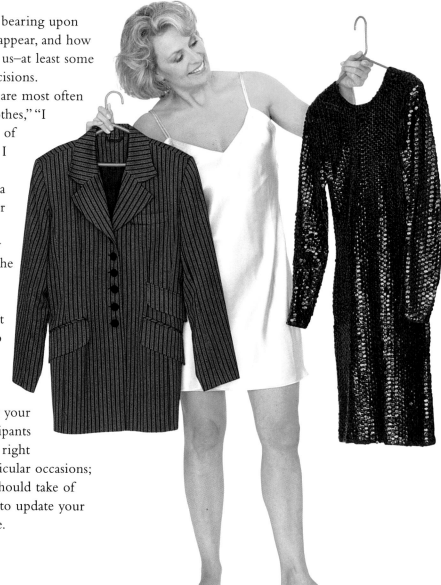

What you wear has an enormous bearing upon how you feel, how young you appear, and how others think of you. Yet almost all of us—at least some of the time—don't make the right decisions.

Here are some of the reasons that are most often quoted: "I've no time to shop for clothes," "I can't afford expensive clothes, or lots of them," "It doesn't really matter what I wear anymore," and "I'm hopeless at choosing clothes for myself; I've got a wardrobe full of mistakes so I'd rather wear what I feel comfortable with," "I'm not sure of the right 'look' now that I'm middle-aged; fashion is for the young."

In truth, you can get away with a lot at 25 that you can't at 50, but that is no reason to give up and decide to live in leggings and baggy sweaters, or perhaps to get into the frumpy grannie look once past 40.

This workshop is all about finding your own style. Using our 10-week participants as models, we'll help you choose the right color for you, the right look for particular occasions; we'll discuss how much notice you should take of current fashions, and show you how to update your wardrobe without spending a fortune.

Finding your new look

If you've lost some weight, toned yourself up, treated yourself to a new hair-do, don't spoil everything by carrying on in the same frumpy skirts and tops or tatty jeans and sweatshirts. Now is the time to treat yourself to some new clothes. But first, before you rush out to start buying, you need to consider some facts that will help prevent you from the buying disasters you've undoubtedly had in the past!

Ceril says, "The first thing to consider is what you actually *want* from your clothes. For all of us, the first priority is to fit our clothes to our lifestyle. As an extreme example, I've known women blow a hard-earned $750 on a high-fashion gown they will wear only once, and then feel guilty about buying decent casual clothes they can wear every weekend."

Think hard before buying any item. Will you get use out of it? Does it fit in with the way you live?

"Next," says Ceril, "Consider what you look good in. The pages that follow give advice on choosing the right colors, styles, and materials for you, and Workshop 10 shows how to dress to flatter your body. So make sure anything you buy fits these simple criteria.

"Then you need to ask yourself, 'Is it easy to wear?'.

Anything you don't feel comfortable in is unlikely to be worn often. Move around in the garment, watch yourself sit in it, walk in it. Raise your arms over your head in it. Is it a good fit? "If you feel it 'wears easy' then you'll enjoy wearing it.'

"It will also help if the item you choose will team with other things in your existing wardrobe (unless you really are starting from scratch, in which case you still need to buy things that can be mixed and matched). Often really nice garments remain unworn simply because they don't fit in well with what you already have, and that includes accessories. Bear this in mind, if choosing a color that's new for you."

If you follow all these tips you don't need to worry too much about whether an outfit is the right one for your age. But just in case you're still not sure, on pages 81 and 82 you'll discover if there is such a thing as an unsuitable look for an age, and just how much of a slave to current fashion trends you should be.

Creating the right image for yourself is as much about thought, balance, and confidence as it is about money and time.

Color Confidence

Read Color Confidence on page 78, then check below to determine your color season.

SUMMER

Summer skin has pink-blue undertones. Usually fair and pale with hair ranging from very blonde to ash or brown, with auburn tones or gray. Eyes are soft gray or pale.

Summer colors – pastel pink and blue-pink, raspberry, blue-red, burgundy, maroon, light lemon-yellow, plum, lavender, mauve, soft white, rose-beige, light-to-medium blue-grays, grayed navy, clear or gray-toned blues, aqua, light-to-dark blue-greens.

NO orange, gold, black.

WINTER

Winter skin also has pink-blue undertones. Most winters are dark-haired and have gray-ish-beige or sallow complexions. Winter eyes are deeper in color than summer eyes.

Winter colors – mostly clear bright colors, light and dark blue-toned pinks, clear and bright reds, blue-red, clear yellow, royal purple, icy violet, white, taupe, gray, black, navy, bright blue and ice blue, bright turquoise, clear bright green.

NO orange, gold.

SPRING

Skin has golden undertones. Some springs may have ivory skin with freckles, others clear, creamy skin. Even with freckles, skin is always clear and bright and skin may tan easily. Eyes are usually clear with golden flecks.

Spring colors – light orange, apricot, peach, salmon, coral, light rust, peachy pink, clear and orange-reds, clear gold, golden-yellow, violet, ivory, creamy beige, camel, light warm gray, golden brown, tan, light clear navy, most clear blues, turquoise, aqua, clear pastel to bright yellow-greens.

NO black, burgundy.

AUTUMN

Skin has golden undertones, with red or auburn hair, with ruddy, or dark golden skin. Autumns with light eyes will look better in the muted autumn colors.

Autumn colors – orange, deep peach, salmon, rust, terracotta, orangy and dark reds, gold, yellow-gold, creamy gold, gold-beige, camel, brown, blue, turquoise, green.

NO pink, burgundy, purple, gray, black.

COLOR CONFIDENCE

or life beyond black leggings...

So you're in a clothes rut. Because it's easy, you always opt for black (or another dark neutral color) and, because it's easy, you opt for leggings and a top. With the help of participants Angela, Sal, Hilary, and Linda, we'll look at some more flattering alternatives.

When you put on an outfit in a color that suits you, wonderful things happen–you look better. . . you look younger. . . you even look healthier. . . your skin tone comes alive. . . and your eyes sparkle. When you put a color near your face that *doesn't* suit you, the reverse happens. So what suits you?

You figure black suits you. After all, it's slimming, isn't it? And it always has suited you, hasn't it? Well, sadly, black is one of the few colors that suit very few older women. You may look slim and smart in it, but there are more flattering colors for you that will also make you look slim and smart.

To find your own best colors, try the "season" test. Ceril explains: "Although it isn't an exact science, most of us can be categorized into one of the four seasons, depending upon the color and tone of our hair, eyes, and skin (see previous page). See if you can work out which season you are. Find a selection of materials in the colors that fit into the category you think you may be and hold them up to your face. If the colors bring your face alive, then you are that season. Most people can wear colors from other seasons and some may look all right. Indeed some people are a mix of more than one season, but this system is a good starting point. Within your color season, you will find some colors you prefer to others, and preference is, of course, important. You can wear colors outside your season (even black!) if you wear them with one of your own colors near your face."

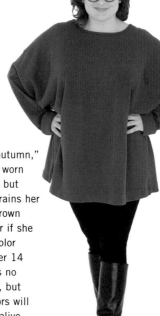

Although an "autumn," Sal has always worn almost nothing but black, which drains her face. A deep brown would be better if she wants a dark color (having lost over 14 pounds, there's no need, though!), but lighter fall colors will bring her face alive.

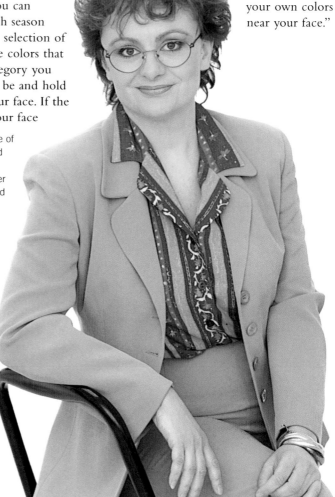

Pale blue is one of Sal's really good colors–her face sparkles and her eyes really stand out.

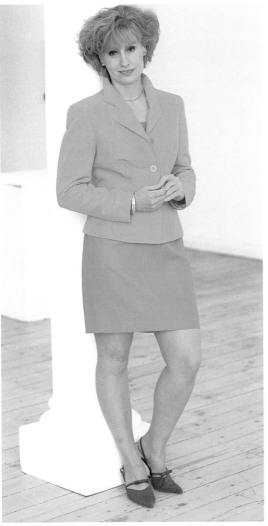

Hilary is a "spring," but tends to live in drab browns and rarely wears bright colors. The moment we put this coral suit on her she looked fantastic and her personality began to bubble, too. This is one of spring's best colors.

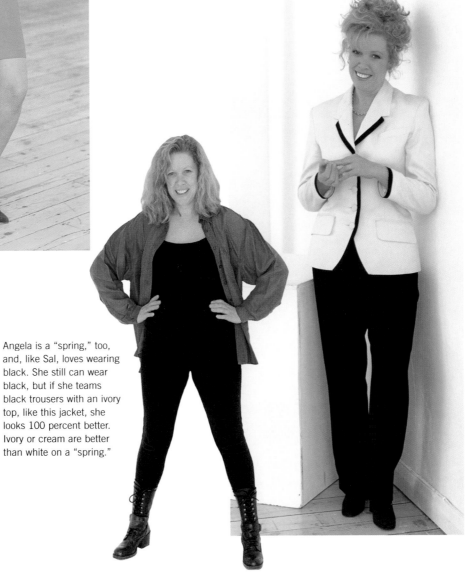

Angela is a "spring," too, and, like Sal, loves wearing black. She still can wear black, but if she teams black trousers with an ivory top, like this jacket, she looks 100 percent better. Ivory or cream are better than white on a "spring."

CASUAL CHIC

Over the last ten years, leggings have changed from being the streetwise uniform of teenagers to the unchic uniform of middle-aged women who think they look wonderful but rarely do. Even leggings worn well are passé and date you more accurately than wrinkles ever could. The baggy sweater that usually tops them hides a good figure or makes an out-of-shape figure look even worse.

*And you would never wear
leggings with high-heel shoes, would you?*

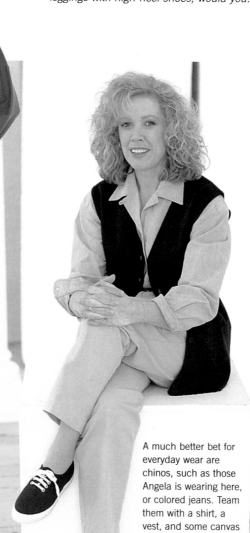

A much better bet for everyday wear are chinos, such as those Angela is wearing here, or colored jeans. Team them with a shirt, a vest, and some canvas sneakers or leather loafers for a much more up-to-date look.

DRESSING FOR YOUR AGE

Every woman has a fear of dressing too young for her age. To my mind, however, just as bad is the woman who insists upon wearing dowdy clothes the moment she hits 50.

There is a fine line between dressing to look younger gracefully, and looking foolish in clothes that are far too young for you. But very few women do, in fact, opt for a young and girlish look. Most, fearing an obvious young look more than anything, go the other way instead, and wear really drab and frumpy clothes long before they need. (In fact, there is *never* a need.) With the help of Linda and Angela, who both do some modeling, we'll examine the old chestnut of "dressing for your age." We'll run through some clothes considerations and point out a few of the mistakes you're likely to make. The comments are only a guide– adapt them to suit your own personality, age, lifestyle, and so on.

Colors and materials

Too young: mixing lots of different brights; plastic, rubber, some leathers.
Too old: all beige; all black; dull, dowdy prints; terry cloth (except for sport).

Skirt lengths and styles

Too young: extremely short; extremely tight.
Too old: mid-calf length; gathered; voluminous; tailored pleats.

Evening wear

Too young: strapless gowns exposing flabby arms/neck/back (OK if you're very well-toned, but check out back view!); too much cleavage showing; flounces and frills.
Too old: scarves used to cover the bits mentioned above (everyone knows that trick).

Casual

Too young: short shorts (unless your legs are perfect and you're on vacation); see-throughs (not wonderful on any age); going bare-legged with anything other than slacks or long skirts (unless your legs are perfect and/or you're on vacation).
Too old: tweedy baggy country look (unless roaming your estate); cardigan; fussy printed polyester dresses.

Accessories

Too young: very high heels; huge platforms; white shoes; baseball caps; Doc Marten/ Caterpillar-type boots unless walking/gardening or similar (Timberlands are OK with a casual outfit); plastic anything.
Too old: frumpy shoes; slippers; head scarves tied under your chin.

Dressing too young

Angela models how not to do it. Her suit fails on several counts: the dress neckline is a bit too low; the skirt a bit too high and much too tight. The jacket is also too tight where it buttons. The lime color, while very trendy at the time Angela modeled, is rendered "over the top" by the addition of the fuchsia detail.

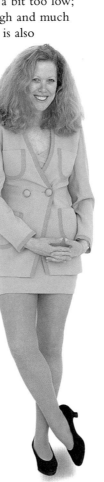

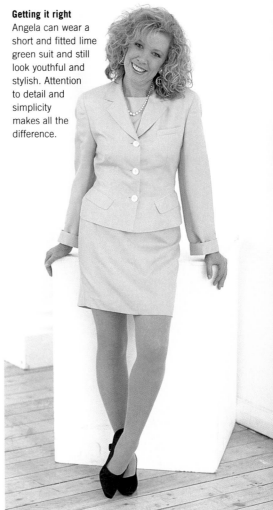

Getting it right
Angela can wear a short and fitted lime green suit and still look youthful and stylish. Attention to detail and simplicity makes all the difference.

Dressing too old

Believe it or not, this is Angela again, all dressed up for the office or a semiformal lunch–and making herself look 20 years older than she is! The drab color of the blouse is completely wrong for the suit and for Angela. The suit skirt is very aging, with its pleats and mid-calf length. The shape of the shoes is way out of date. The complete outfit is shapeless, and the aging, harsh hairline and pearls reinforce the dowdy effect.

Getting it right
It is possible to look neat and efficient and young, too! Here Angela wears a simple straight-skirted belted coat dress and some up-to-date shoes. A less severe hairstyle finishes the look very well.

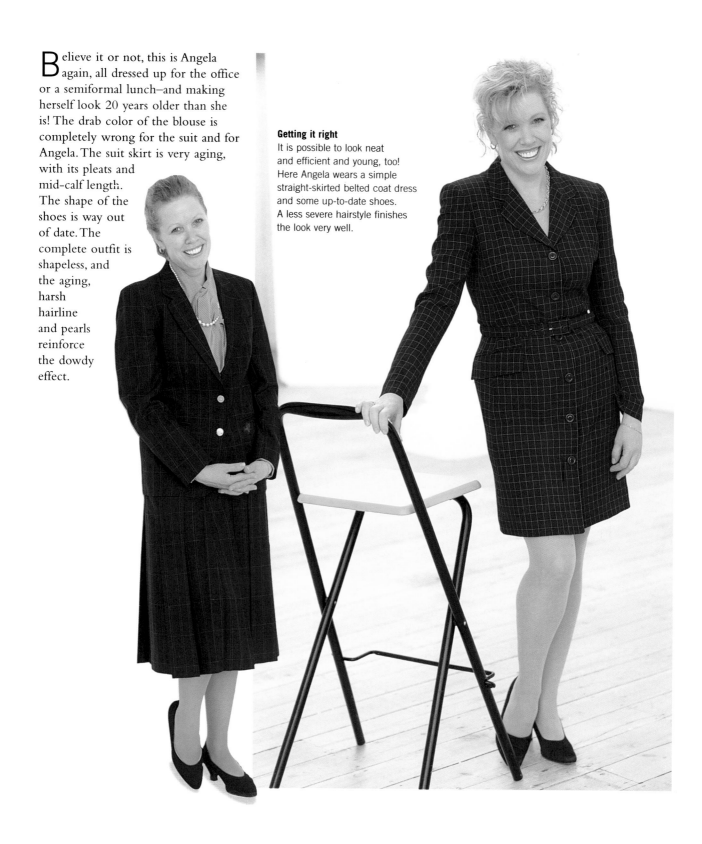

Dressing too frumpy

Linda owns this dress but brought it along to our studio knowing it to be a terrible mistake! Avoid, at all costs, polyester printed dresses with self belts, pleats, or gathers and ending at mid-calf. Avoid loud prints and sleeves that finish around the elbow. All will conspire to make you look like a fashion dinosaur and twice your age.

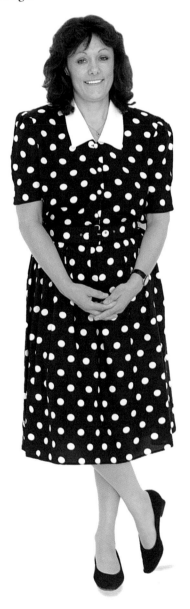

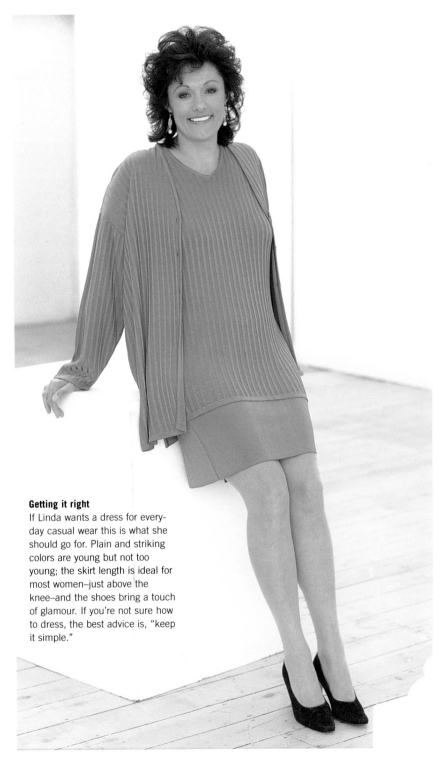

Getting it right
If Linda wants a dress for every-day casual wear this is what she should go for. Plain and striking colors are young but not too young; the skirt length is ideal for most women–just above the knee–and the shoes bring a touch of glamour. If you're not sure how to dress, the best advice is, "keep it simple."

WARDROBE WORKOUT

Sue is a part-time family physician and a mother of two. Having paid little attention to her clothes since giving birth to her oldest daughter, now eight, Sue was desperate for some practical style suggestions. Sue, 39, had put on 14 pounds since having children and, largely because of this extra weight, hadn't bothered about her clothes for years.

Her wardrobe was full of dowdy mid-length skirts and sensible pullovers and cardigans—her typical style during office hours. Colors were dark, muted, or white. Ceril says, "The outfit [left] is typical of the kind of thing Sue has been wearing for years. A safe and nondescript skirt with a knitted cardigan that makes her look much larger than she really is (a neat size 10 in this photo). The skirt length, opaque tights, and old-fashioned flat shoes finish a dowdy image that doesn't flatter Sue at all! Sue has chosen clothes that don't stand out—nothing to show off her figure."

"But," says Sue, "I have little confidence in what to buy for myself now. I know I need a new look, but I'd rather not spend too much money on any single item."

"Sue is a 'summer' person," says Ceril. "She is going to look really good in icy pastels, and in bright shades of blue and green, and bluish red. The muted, drab colors are making her fade away. The colors I suggest will really bring her look alive and bring out her true personality.

"Sue has lost 14 pounds in the 10 weeks, and also needs to rethink the shape of her clothes. She is quite small at 5 foot 4 inches and longer length and baggy skirts and fussy knits swamp her. She is ideal for above-the-knee straight skirts, rather than the longer length she has preferred, and

At home or for holidays, Sue really does suit these bright greens and blues in easy-care, easy-wear fabrics.

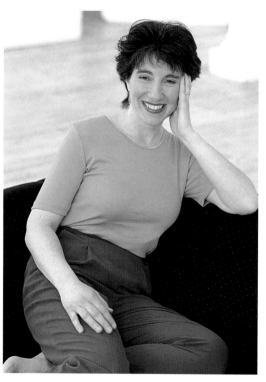

hip-length jackets. Lighter shoes and pantyhose—and a little makeup—will all help to lift her look."

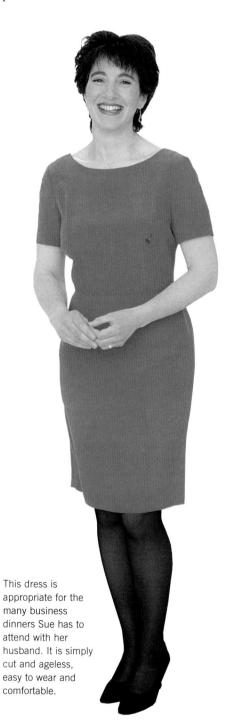

This dress is appropriate for the many business dinners Sue has to attend with her husband. It is simply cut and ageless, easy to wear and comfortable.

Sue loved this suit, which is surprisingly inexpensive. If clothes are kept simple, you can get away with not spending a fortune. "I am going to buy a couple of simple suits and wear them to work instead of my jumpers and skirts!" says Sue.

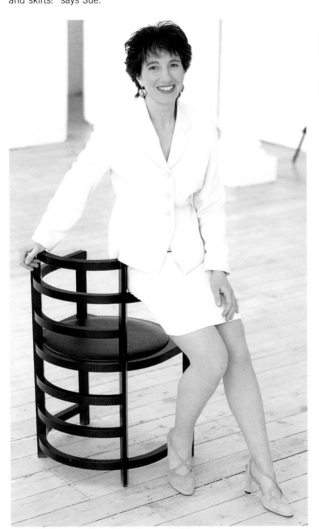

REVAMP YOUR WARDROBE

Give your own wardrobe a workout. Allow as long as you need for each part of this exercise.

Part One

Go through absolutely everything in your current wardrobe, putting it all into one of four of the following piles and remember everything Ceril has taught you about style:

1 Things you wear and that pass the style test.

2 Things that you never wear and/or are not flattering. Give this pile away.

3 Things that may have possibilities if you can find items to team with them.

4 Things that need mending/shortening/taking in or other alterations.

Do the same with your shoes, bags, belts, etc., teaming up accessories with suitable outfits from pile 1 and throwing out everything that really isn't going to be worn any more.

Determine the gaps in your wardrobe (bearing in mind your own lifestyle) by checking this list of items that will be most useful:

● At least two or three good, classic items (suits, pants suit, and dress and jacket combinations) you can wear frequently and maybe pair the jackets or pants or skirts with other items.

● Several bolder, smaller items to enliven the classics–shirts, vests, sweaters, and tunics.

● Several casual mix-and-matches for everyday wear–chinos and jeans, with matching tops.

● One or two outfits suitable for evening–separates allow more flexibility.

● Accessories to match all these outfits.

Now write a list of what you need to fill the gaps. If you've lost or gained a lot of weight and/or haven't shopped for ages, the gaps may be quite large but you can always build up a new wardrobe slowly or, if you're so inclined, check out one of the many excellent consignment stores for low-cost quality items. Don't be afraid to buy inexpensive small high-fashion items–T-shirts in this season's color, for instance, which will update and enliven your wardrobe considerably.

Part Two

Allow as long as you need for this exercise, which is a shopping trip!

It's time to go and try on as many things as you can (preferably alone . . . your own judgment is something you need to learn to trust) in as many stores as you can. (Take spare shoes, pantyhose, and a T-shirt with you if intending to try various styles–the wrong accessories with an outfit can distract you from the right decision.) A mall with a big department store and lots of smaller stores within it is an excellent location. Try, try, try. If an item passes the six-point checklist below, consider adding it to your wardrobe:

● Does it fit?

● Does the color suit you?

● Does the style suit you?

● Does it go with other things in your wardrobe?

● Will you get plenty of use from it?

● Do you really like it?

*F ew women-even most of the supermodels-have perfect figures.
In this workshop, Ceril Campbell makes the most of a variety of figure
shapes-and shows you what to avoid.*

10 STYLE ASSESSMENT 2
DRESSING FOR YOUR SHAPE

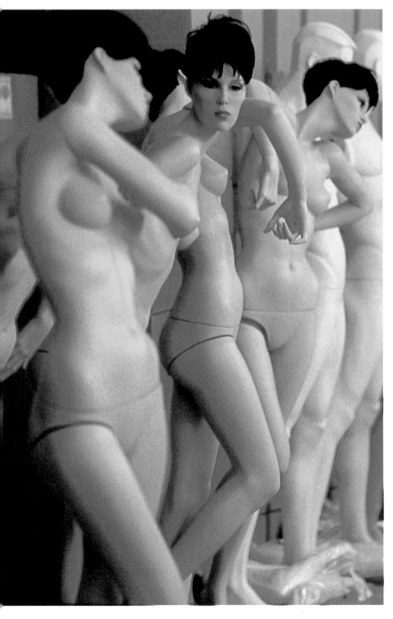

B y the time we reach the 30s and 40s, most of us know only too well which features of our bodies we dislike. Even with careful diet and plenty of toning exercise, basic body shape is something you have to live with. But, with the clever use of clothes—and that includes design, color, material, length, and so on—to draw attention *away* from your worst features and *toward* your good points, you can make yourself look better proportioned.

Incredible, then, that many of us actually do the reverse—often choosing clothes that make us look *worse* than we really are. So next time you go shopping, take a few minutes to look hard at each outfit you try on and ask yourself, is it really flattering to your figure, or could you do better?

Over the next seven pages, you'll see some of our 10-week participants modeling outfits that don't suit their figures at all (often things they had bought themselves), and we'll tell you why. Then we put them into something much more flattering and again we'll tell you why. Using these examples, plus the tips you'll find on each page, you won't make the same mistakes.

I hope you'll be inspired to go through your wardrobe and throw out those clothes that are not doing your body any favors, right away!

HILARY
minimizing hips and thighs

Hilary has an excellent figure but, because her bust is quite small and her thighs are heavy compared with her upper body, she tends to look "hippy" in some outfits.

If you're pear-shaped:

DO

• Wear small shoulder pads to balance out your body.
• Wear darker colors on the lower body.
• Wear solid colors on the lower body.
• Wear vertical seams or stripes on the lower body.
• Wear shaped, not straight-cut, long-line jackets to cover the hips and thighs.
• Wear tapered, slim-legged pants that skim over the thighs.

DON'T

• Wear bulky fabrics on the lower body.
• Wear tops that fall on the widest part of your hips or thighs.
• Wear belts too tight around the waist; this will make hips look bigger.

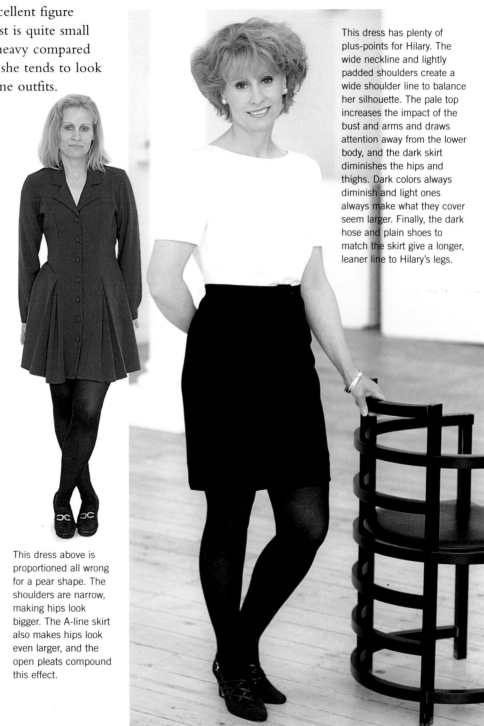

This dress above is proportioned all wrong for a pear shape. The shoulders are narrow, making hips look bigger. The A-line skirt also makes hips look even larger, and the open pleats compound this effect.

This dress has plenty of plus-points for Hilary. The wide neckline and lightly padded shoulders create a wide shoulder line to balance her silhouette. The pale top increases the impact of the bust and arms and draws attention away from the lower body, and the dark skirt diminishes the hips and thighs. Dark colors always diminish and light ones always make what they cover seem larger. Finally, the dark hose and plain shoes to match the skirt give a longer, leaner line to Hilary's legs.

PAMELA
a typical apple

Pamela, like many women in their late 40s, 50s, and 60s, is an apple shape with a large waist and tummy, and slim arms and legs.

When this photo was taken, Pam had already lost more than 3 inches from around her waist, but this shirtwaist dress (her own) adds more inches than she'd taken off! It's also the kind of dress no woman of any age should consider wearing! The print is unflattering; the dark belt draws attention to the stomach; the slightly blouson top adds inches at each side of her waist, and the pleats hanging straight from the waist make her look wide all the way down. The dowdy length skirt completes the unflattering picture.

Apple shapes should skim over their middles with well-cut clothes that give long, clean unfussy lines. This tweed pants suit makes Pam look 10 pounds lighter–and 20 years younger. Neutral colors can be very glamorous if they are worn in the right way, and there is no need to discount wearing a pants suit whatever your age. If you find the waistband tight, select suits with some stretch in the waist-band–there are plenty available. The silk T-shirt worn over the pants is a better bet for apples than a top worn tucked in; and the slim legs and arms of this suit add to the slim lines.

If you're apple-shaped:

DO:
- Keep details around the waist to a minimum.
- Create slightly angular lines to your outline with light shoulder pads or tailored shoulders and open placket jackets, straight skirts or straight-legged slacks.
- Wear tunic-style tops over slacks and skirts, rather than tuck them in.
- Wear short skirts to show off slim legs.

DON'T:
- Wear loose-pleated skirts; pick stitched pleats instead.
- Wear gathered skirts.
- Wear pockets anywhere near the waistline.
- Wear jodhpurs if you have thin legs and a big stomach.
- Wear wide-legged pants.
- Wear formal suits with waist-length or cropped jackets.

KAY
coping with a big bust

Kay has a 39-inch bust, which can seem even larger because she is relatively slim. She doesn't like her bust and tries to disguise it with baggy tops and blouses. A tailored look is a better approach.

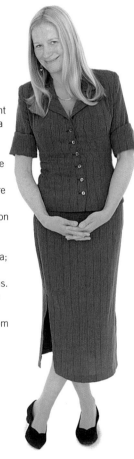

If you like your bust and want to show it off, this could be a good outfit, but for Kay, it isn't. It accentuates her top-heavy shape because the jacket is too tight and is straining at the buttons; there is a horizontal seam across the bustline, drawing attention to it. The sleeves end at the lower line of the bust, drawing attention to that area; and the waisted jacket also makes the bust more obvious. The long skirt covers up the asset that Kay should be using to detract attention from her upper body–those long, long legs!

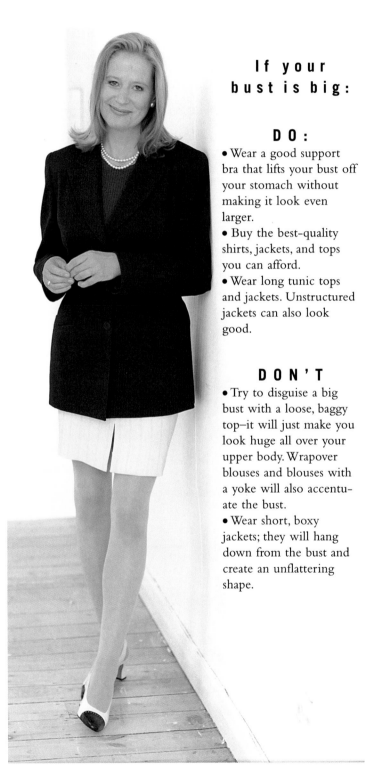

Kay couldn't have done better if this suit had been especially designed for her. The dark navy, well-cut jacket skims over her bustline and the solid camisole underneath creates a simple, understated line to the whole upper body area. The eye is drawn to the pale short skirt and to Kay's legs–exactly the effect we wanted to achieve.

If your bust is big:

DO:
• Wear a good support bra that lifts your bust off your stomach without making it look even larger.
• Buy the best-quality shirts, jackets, and tops you can afford.
• Wear long tunic tops and jackets. Unstructured jackets can also look good.

DON'T
• Try to disguise a big bust with a loose, baggy top–it will just make you look huge all over your upper body. Wrapover blouses and blouses with a yoke will also accentuate the bust.
• Wear short, boxy jackets; they will hang down from the bust and create an unflattering shape.

SALLY
tall dressing for petites

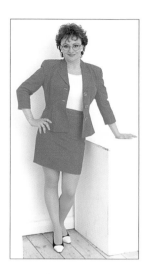

Sal has a nice curvy figure, she's 5 foot 3 inches, with a short body. But she wants advice on dressing for those curves and wants to look taller.

Sal wears a lot of black, and thought this suit would look good on her –but it's a disaster! The short jacket cuts her body in two and makes it look too boxy. Sal has a good waist and the boxy cut loses it. The double breast and heavy lapel detail does nothing for her bustline, except make her look bulky. The shoulders are too heavy and wide for Sal, and the polo neck accentuates Sal's short neck. The wide sleeves swamp Sal and add width, too. The short skirt forms another box shape, compounding the problem.

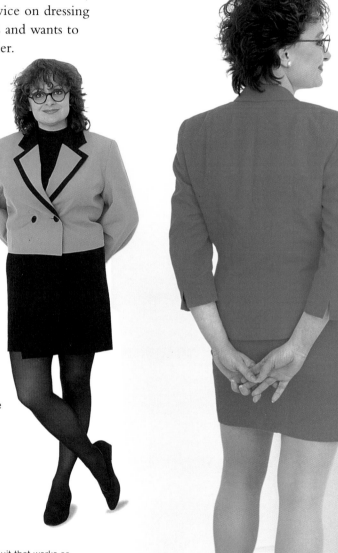

This is a similar type of suit that works so much better. Here's why. It's all one color (if you take one color through an outfit, it will always make you look taller and slimmer). The jacket sets off Sal's curves, and is slightly longer and single-breasted, slimming Sal's upper body, particularly her bust. The narrow sleeves suit Sal much better, and the little white low-necked blouse elongates her neck and diminishes her jawline. Isn't it amazing how two outfits so similar in intention can produce such contrasting images?

If you're short and curvy:

DO:
• Go for one main color from head to toe; with hose and shoes that match each other, too.
• Go for slim skirts and fitted jackets that follow your curves.
• Wear slim pants and mid-heel shoes.

DON'T:
• Wear voluminous clothes; they will over-power you.
• Wear large patterns; they will have the same effect.
• Wear long skirts.
• Wear very high heels — they will make you look out of proportion.

LINDA
dressing slim while dieting

Linda has lost more than 15 pounds on our 10-week program, but still has some more to lose. She wants advice for dressing slim in the meantime!

This dress is out of Linda's wardrobe–but she admits it's not her style! Linda is a size 16-18, with big bust, waist, hips, and thighs. This dress manages to get it all wrong for someone of Linda's size. It has an unflattering neckline and the cutaway sleeves are not good if your upper arms are a bit flabby (something that can happen over 40, however slim you are). The white belt draws attention to the waist and tummy area and also to a droopy bust. (Linda needs a better bra.) The lightly gathered skirt makes her midriff look larger than it is–and those bright horizontal stripes are a no-no for any body area you want to slim down. The length of the dress is decidedly frumpy and hides Linda's slim calves.

Whoever said larger women can't wear fitted clothes? Linda looks 30 pounds lighter than in her "before" picture, with this terrific ensemble of black crewneck fine-knit sweater, single-breasted jacket in fine black stripes on pale beige, with stretch jodhpurs to match, all finished with a pair of black jodhpur boots.

This is the exception to the rule. Pale colors enlarge and dark ones diminish. In this instance the pale beige doesn't have that effect because Linda's coloring really suits paler colors. The dark buttons draw the eye to the center; the jacket is very well cut and neatly covers Linda's bottom, and the jodhpurs show off her slim calves and ankles.

If you're plump:

DO:
• Go for plain materials rather than wild patterns.
• Choose vertical stripes.
• Choose fine materials rather than heavy ones – select thin knits, not textured ones; silk, not satin; linen, not terry cloth, and so on.
• Go for casually tailored styles.

DON'T:
• Wear long flowing garments in bold patterns.
• Wear shiny fabrics.
• Wear clothes that are too tight.
• Wear puff sleeves or ruffles.

SUE
Long lines for short waists

Sue has a lovely figure, but a short waist. When we first met her she was wearing almost everything that is exactly wrong for a short waist—especially if, like Sue, you aren't very tall.

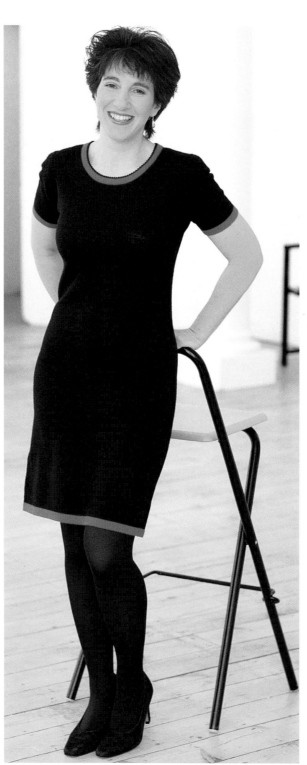

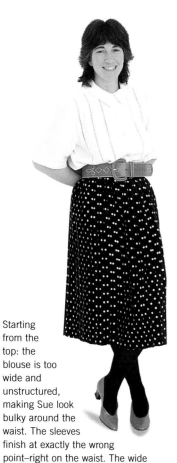

Starting from the top: the blouse is too wide and unstructured, making Sue look bulky around the waist. The sleeves finish at exactly the wrong point—right on the waist. The wide bright belt draws attention to the waist and shortens it further. The gathered skirt flaring from under the belt adds another bulky layer. For a taller women, the skirt length would not be too bad, but it makes Sue look even shorter. The shoes, which don't match the hose, shorten the overall look, too.

If you're petite and short-waisted:

DO:
- Wear shift dresses.
- Wear single-breasted jackets to hip length (no longer).
- Wear empire-line or drop-waist dresses.
- Keep lines simple.
- Wear tunic tops with long, narrow pants.

DON'T:
- Wear blouses and skirts.
- Wear wide stiff belts—a narrow, fluid hipster belt is a good choice if you have to belt up.
- Wear gathered skirts or blouses without darts (unless worn outside slacks or skirts).
- Wear fussy clothes.

Although navy isn't one of Sue's own best colors, it does suit most women (if this dark navy isn't perfect, then a lighter French navy would be an alternative). This simple dress shows off Sue's figure. It skims over her waist, creating a long, lean line. The length is much better for her, and the low, rounded neckline draws attention to her face rather than the waist. The master touch of red trimming at the neck and hem takes the eye up, then down. It never lingers around the middle, as it did on Sue's "before" outfit.

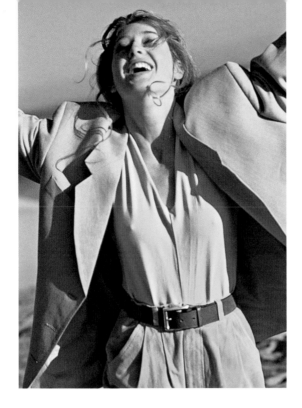

ENERGY SOURCES

The Vital You

Energy. . . vitality. . . sparkle – the missing ingredients in so many women's lives. And yet an abundance of energy, both mental and physical, *is* the master key to a fulfilling life because it has a profound effect upon what you do, how you feel, and how you look. Think back to ten or twenty years ago when it was normal for you to wake up refreshed and alert, keen to get up and on with the day; when you looked forward to what lay ahead; felt excited by challenges, and packed more into a day than you sometimes do now in a week.

Now your 'norm' is to wake up reluctantly and wish you could spend the day in bed with the phone off the hook – even a good book is too much effort to read. If only you could get back that youthful joie de vivre; if only you could look in the mirror and see bright-eyed enthusiasm. But, sadly, loss of vitality is just part of getting older, isn't it? You slow down, lose your edge.

There are two keys to getting your vitality back. The first is in embracing the energy-givers. From what you eat to how you breathe, from learning to relax to planning your days better and getting your body fit to cope–you need to use the energy givers to empower you.

The second is in clearing your life of the things that drain your energy–the physical and emotional factors that are bringing you down. Minor ailments, bore-dom, poor sleep patterns, overwork, and poor nutrition are just a few of the issues. This second section of the book aims to help you do both. The real, pure feeling of zest for life–of feeling in control again–is something you can't fake, but when you've got it is guaranteed to melt the years away.

*I*f you lack energy, the first thing you need to do is check out your general health. Many physical problems can deplete energy, if only because "it's one more thing to worry about."

HEALTH CHECK

Go through the health checklist, opposite, and every time you check a symptom, refer to the Action column for what to do. Many of the symptoms are covered in other workshops to which you'll be guided; for others you'll find recommended courses of action, or it will be suggested you see the appropriate doctor. Don't ignore symptoms that need a professional examination! For example, about 10 percent of unexplained chronic fatigue cases are due to an illness that has gone undetected, such as thyroid problems, rheumatism, anemia, or diabetes. After all, you value your own body more than you value your car—don't you?

Eight simple ways to a healthier you

❶ Complete physical once a year including pelvic exam and Pap test

❷ Don't smoke

❸ Moderate your alcohol consumption, if you drink

❹ Sleep, rest, and relaxation

❺ Fresh air

❻ Regular exercise

❼ Healthy diet, healthy weight

❽ Enjoy life

Health Checklist

Check the symptoms that relate to you under every section:

Symptom	Action

Stress-related symptoms

❏ Disrupted eating patterns	Workshop 13
❏ Digestive problems	See your doctor; Workshop 13
❏ Insomnia	See family doctor; Workshops 15–17
❏ Fatigue not linked to insomnia	Workshops 13–15 and 17–24; see family doctor
❏ Recurrent minor infections	See family doctor
❏ Palpitations/breathlessness	See family doctor
❏ Depression/crying/fear/panic	See family doctor or counselor; Workshops 14–24
❏ Irritability/aggression	See family doctor; Workshops 14–24
❏ Lack of concentration/memory	See family doctor; Workshops 14–16
❏ Loss of interest in sex/social life	See family doctor; Workshops 21, 22; refer to sex symptoms section below

Sex symptoms

❏ Premenstrual syndrome	See family doctor and/or gynecologist; Workshop 13; regular exercise, use natural diuretics, such as celery, fennel, lettuce, melon, citrus, tomatoes, parsley
❏ Heavy/prolonged/frequent/ painful periods	See family doctor or gynecologist; consider hormone replacement therapy
❏ Painful intercourse	See family doctor or gynecologist; consider hormone replacement therapy; try lubricant
❏ Lack of sex drive	See family doctor and/or gynecologist and/or counselor at end of 10 weeks if no improvement; Workshops 12–16, 21, 22, 24;

Aches and pains

❏ Back/neck pain	See family doctor and/or osteopath; Workshops 3, 4; check chairs, bed, driving position
❏ Headaches	See family doctor; Workshops 13, 15
❏ Joint pain	See family doctor for suitable treatment; exercise; and diet; Workshop 4
❏ Toothache	See dentist

Frequent minor illnesses

❏ Colds	Workshops 13, 14; take extra vitamin C and zinc
❏ Sore throat	See family doctor
❏ Sore/red eyes	See family doctor; take extra vitamin C; consider allergy
❏ Irregular bowel movements	See family doctor; Workshops 13, 15
❏ Candida (yeast infection)	See family doctor and/or gynecologist
❏ Cystitis	See family doctor; drink plenty of water

Menopause plus

❏ Hot flashes	See family doctor and/or gynecologist; consider taking hormone replacement therapy, vitamin E supplements
❏ Sleeplessness	Workshops 15–17
❏ Lack of sex drive	See sex symptom section above
❏ Fatigue	See family doctor; Workshops 12-16 and all of Section 3;
❏ Weight gain	Workshop 2, then 13
❏ Stress incontinence	See family doctor; pelvic floor exercise; and diet; also Workshop 4

10 symptoms you should never ignore

❶ Chest pains on exertion

❷ Unexplained weight loss or gain

❸ Unexplained pain anywhere in body lasting more than a few days

❹ Unexplained fatigue continuing for more than a week after trying all remedies suggested left

❺ Changes in moles or the appearance of new ones

❻ Internal bleeding other than menstruation

❼ Breast lumps

❽ Constant headache

❾ Unexplained fainting/dizziness

❿ Nausea/sickness lasting more than a day or two

*M*ost of us underestimate the importance of thoughtful management of our own time. Yet with streamlining strategies and sensible planning and control, the extra time you buy yourself can make all the difference to your energy level and your life.

WORKSHOP 12 TIME MANAGEMENT

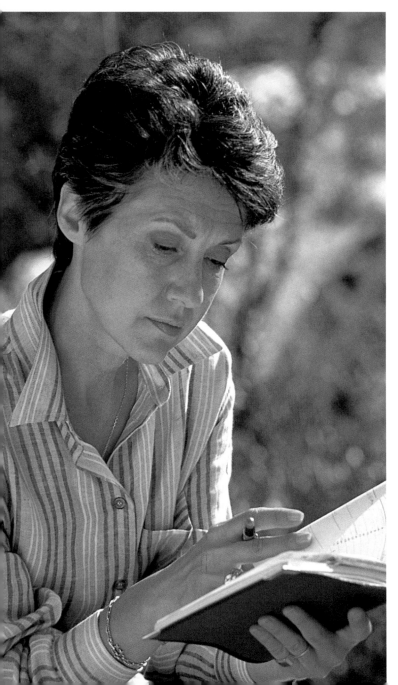

We all waste time, even when we think we don't, and cutting down that waste is vital for women who often have to pack more into their days than the average man. I don't know one woman for whom "finding time" *isn't* a never-ending problem.

The "busy-busy syndrome," with life always half an hour behind schedule; with long, long hours and never any time for yourself means you are living in a permanently stressful, energy-draining state. Creating extra time with the help of some simple strategies means stress levels go down, energy increases—and you're on the way to getting the life you want.

Your Time Diary

First, keep your own "time diary" for three days.

● Make two columns: 1. *time*; 2. *what you did*; leave room for a third column which will remain blank for now.

● List everything you do from the time you wake to going to sleep. Obviously, keeping the diary is going to take up some of your precious time, but it will be time well spent.

● Carry on with the workshop and fill in the blank column afterward.

Monday 7.15 am
7.35 am
8.00 am

Planning Ahead

It is hard to manage time efficiently without lists. If you already live by lists, make sure yours really work for you.

You need a "to do today" list–ideally broken up into professional life and personal life. And you need a "to do this week" list. I also like a "long-term" list, but that's optional.

Write your "today" list the night before (it will help you sleep well). In the morning go through your list and ruthlessly cross out anything that isn't really necessary and/or you don't really want to do. For this, you need to get into the habit of setting priorities. Also, Parkinson's Law dictates that a job will expand to fill the time available. Rather than have this happen to you, allot the time each item on your list should take, then try to stick to it.

Every day, work through your list from the top. Aim to get through the list in all but the most unexpected circumstances. At the end of the day, make the list for the following day, including anything that you didn't do that day. If, after two weeks, an item is still on the list and still not done, either do it immediately or take it off the list and forget it.

Two other kinds of lists worth making:

TV List–If you want to limit how much time you spend watching television, go through the viewing for the week ahead and make a note of anything you really want to watch (ask yourself *why* you want to watch it) and don't watch anything else.

Menu List–particularly if you have to cook for people other than yourself. Always plan meals on a weekly basis and shop after you've done your list. This will prevent last-minute trips to the supermarket every other day You'll save time and energy by having another area of your life settled in advance.

Be Firm

Being firm, both with others and yourself, is perhaps the biggest time-saver of all.

At Work

- If possible, try to limit the amount of overtime you put in, and balance the demands of your job with your own needs.
- Accept that you may not be able to complete each task perfectly but you can always be competent. Perfectionism can be a strain on others as well as on yourself.
- Keep meetings as short as possible by focusing on the subject. If colleagues stray off the point, politely bring them back.
- Delegate whenever appropriate (see page 99).

In Your Personal Life

- Learn to say "no." Never agree to do anything you don't want to do. Sounds simple, but we almost all accept invitations we'd rather refuse, agree to charitable works we don't have time for, let people invite themselves for the weekend even though we don't get along with them all that well. . . you know the drill. You do it because you want to be liked or haven't learned to say no. And are the people making demands the people you want to be liked by, anyway? Isn't it better to like yourself first? Say "no" and start practicing now. Say "no" anyway you like–directly, diplomatically, or with a white lie. But say no!
- Know your limitations–keep your commitments within the bounds of what you can do without exhausting yourself. There is no need to feel guilty about this; it is common sense.

Be Fit

Physical fitness helps you get through almost everything in your life more quickly and efficiently. Being fit means being stronger (so chores are accomplished more easily); being fit means a better supply of oxygen to your brain (so you have better mental alertness to do mental tasks, read quicker, absorb information quicker, and so on); being fit also means less chance of being laid up in bed with illness.

Make sure to use some of the time you save keeping yourself as fit as possible by checking out the stamina workshop on page 105.

Woke up. Listened to news on TV. Got up and got ready. Left home for work (no time for breakfast...)

Could have got ready while listening to news then had time for breakfast.

CASE HISTORY

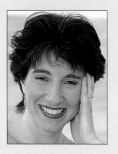

Sue: With two small daughters, a career as a family doctor running a weekday practice, and a house to run with only occasional child care, Sue still manages to find time to spend 1½ days a week studying acupuncture *and* enjoys eating out and socializing.

"I even watch TV in the evenings," she says. "It is my relaxation then, so I don't restrict myself much."

So how does she fit everything in?

"I seem to do much more when everything is busy. You know, if I wake up and realize there is a lot to fit into the day that can't be postponed, then I seem to just get more done.

"I suppose when there really *is* too much to do, it is the housework that suffers, but I feel less guilty about that than I would if I spent less time with the girls (aged eight and five), for instance. You have to get your priorities right for you."

Review Your Sleeping Pattern

Getting enough quality sleep is vital, which is why a workshop is devoted to just that (see Workshop 16 on page 112). However, one in three people stay in bed longer than needed. Ironically, too much sleep can cause a drowsy, headachy feeling. Many people can cut down the time they spend in bed by up to an hour without any ill effects and the benefit of an extra seven hours a week of time. So try these tips for saving bed time:

- Don't go to bed until you are tired.

- Leave a window open a crack. Turn down the heating as low as you find comfortable. Using these strategies you are likely to wake up slightly earlier than usual and feel more refreshed, avoiding the temptation of rolling over and going back to sleep.

- Get up as soon as you wake up; don't linger.

- Set the alarm to wake you 30 minutes earlier than usual for a week. See if notice any difference in how you feel during the day. If you don't feel tired, take another half hour off the following week. You may even feel better.

Be Aware of Time

It is perfectly okay sometimes to do absolutely nothing, as you will find out in Workshop 15. You need to set aside that time on a regular basis and enjoy it; let it revive you. It is also fine to daydream if it helps you plan out what you really want and plot your future. But don't fritter away time—or allow other people to waste time for you.

Here are some examples of time frittered, not well spent:

- Watching TV just because it is on. If you can, move to another room or turn it off. Instead, read or write or work on a hobby, or do something on your list.

- Listening to gossip. Be polite if you meet people you know in the street or in a store but don't feel obliged to stand and chat for ages if you are busy. Be firm, move on.

- Reading gossip. Don't buy tabloids that offer little except showbiz gossip and voyeurism on other people's lives. A good book will teach you more about human nature. Talking of books –I never continue reading a book if, after ten pages, I find it boring. If I want to know the ending, I read the last few pages.

- Listening to telemarketers. If you're not interested in the product, politely say, "No, thank you" and hang up.

- Waiting for people or things. It's surprising how often you find yourself hanging around for 10 minutes or so just waiting. Don't waste it, use it. If you've cooked a supper for friends and everything is ready but they are late, for example, don't just stand in the kitchen checking your watch. Do a 10-minute task on your list or read a few pages of your book. While a pot of water comes to a boil for pasta, throw out any stale food in the refrigerator or make that dental or doctor's appointment you have been putting off. Never go to an appointment or meeting without something to do if you have to wait.

Delegate

Women are often poor at delegating, especially at home. But if you live with a partner and/or children over the age of five, they should all help out. If, for example, there are three other people in the household and each of them spends 20 minutes a day doing chores you used to do, that's a whole hour of your time saved. And, as research indicates that the average woman spends *six* hours a day on home-related tasks, including shopping and cooking, you need to save as much time as you can! If you have spent years not delegating, this new tough line may take some time–and determination–to bring about. But stand firm! It can be done.

Here is the route to follow:

1 Explain that as a family everyone must share household responsibilities. Besides, less work for mother means there will be more time to spend together and a more relaxed atmosphere.

2 Explain what it is they should be doing (e.g. small children picking up their toys, older children doing the dishes, partner ironing own clothes).

3 Remind them now and then.

4 Don't do it yourself.

5 If all else fails, employ paid help and explain to the reluctant helpers that you can no longer afford their designer clothes, fine wine, vacations, or expensive presents they have come to expect because the cash had to be diverted. If you already have paid help, remember to let her/him do the work; there's no need to clean the house for the housekeeper.

Learn Time-Saving Strategies

Sometimes you'll be doing things the same old way out of habit. But a few new tricks will save you time. Here are a few suggestions; think up more of your own:

● Beating a trail around the stores for anything from clothes to plants to presents is a waste of time and energy when almost anything you want can be purchased by telephone, fax, computer, the Internet, or mail and sent virtually anywhere. If you pay by credit card you are protected.

● When possible, cook double batches of soups, stews, and other dishes for the freezer.

● Dress using one color as your signature color. This simplifies coordinating and accesorizing outfits, and saves time deciding what to wear to the office or to pack for vacations.

● Have an easy-care hairstyle.

● Double up as much as you can; don't just see a friend–see a friend *and* go to the art exhibition you have been trying to get to for ages.

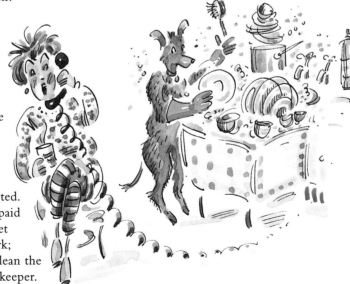

*J*ust as a car needs the right fuel to run efficiently and perform well, so does your body.
The well-fed body is less likely to suffer from mental or physical sluggishness; from fatigue,
minor ailments, colds, and a general feeling of being "under par." Sound eating geared to your own
lifestyle can help your body cope better with the pressures and pace of modern life. So begin
thinking of food as fuel to empower you and enhance your performance, and you
will see just how important it is to eat right for energy.

WORKSHOP 13

EATING FOR ENERGY

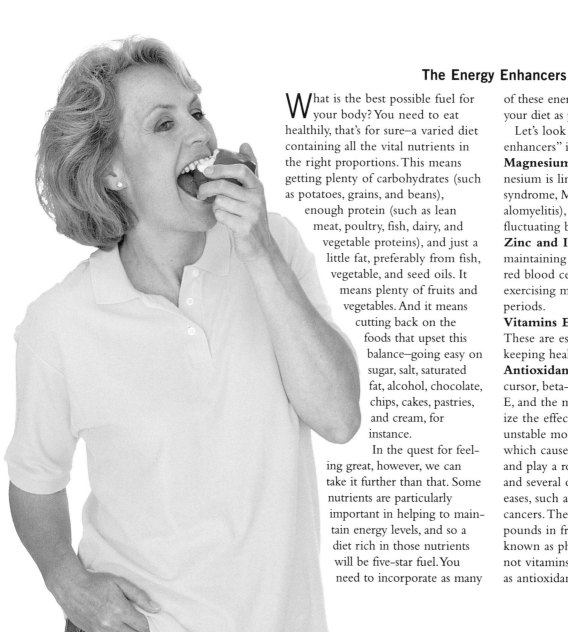

The Energy Enhancers

What is the best possible fuel for your body? You need to eat healthily, that's for sure—a varied diet containing all the vital nutrients in the right proportions. This means getting plenty of carbohydrates (such as potatoes, grains, and beans), enough protein (such as lean meat, poultry, fish, dairy, and vegetable proteins), and just a little fat, preferably from fish, vegetable, and seed oils. It means plenty of fruits and vegetables. And it means cutting back on the foods that upset this balance—going easy on sugar, salt, saturated fat, alcohol, chocolate, chips, cakes, pastries, and cream, for instance.

In the quest for feeling great, however, we can take it further than that. Some nutrients are particularly important in helping to maintain energy levels, and so a diet rich in those nutrients will be five-star fuel. You need to incorporate as many of these energy-enhancing foods into your diet as possible.

Let's look at these "energy enhancers" in detail.

Magnesium. A deficiency of magnesium is linked to chronic fatigue syndrome, ME (myalgic encephalomyelitis), low energy levels, and fluctuating blood sugar levels.

Zinc and Iron. Both are vital for maintaining energy levels and healthy red blood cells, especially if you are exercising more or if you have heavy periods.

Vitamins E and the B group. These are essential for making and keeping healthy red blood cells.

Antioxidants. The vitamin A precursor, beta-carotene, vitamins C and E, and the mineral selenium neutralize the effect of the "free radicals," unstable molecules in our bodies which cause cell and tissue damage and play a role in the aging process and several of the degenerative diseases, such as heart disease and some cancers. There are also many compounds in fresh fruits and vegetables, known as phytochemicals, that are not vitamins or minerals but also act as antioxidants.

An energy-enhancing diet will not only be high in the nutrients and foods we've discussed previously but will also be low in those that have a negative effect on your energy or are of little or no nutritional value.

Alcohol. A glass of wine with your evening meal is fine. A little alcohol can be good for your heart, literally, and good for your soul. But more than a little is not a good idea. Drinking too much alcohol robs your body of the nutrients that are vital for your health and energy. Its effects as a diuretic can lead to dehydration which when combined with alcohol's qualities as a depressant can make you feel tired and cranky.

Sugar. White sugar is the only food that is completely nutrient-deficient apart from the calories it contains. Soda, candy, and other simple sugar foods give very short-term energy boosts, but unless you eat something nutritious shortly after, you will soon feel less energetic and more fatigued than before. The best foods for long-term energy are those that ensure a steady blood sugar level, such as whole grains, fresh vegetables, and lean proteins.

Junk foods. If your diet is high in commercially produced sugary and/or fatty snacks and meals—like potato and corn chips, cakes, cookies, pies, chocolate, other desserts, and candy—your body will suffer. Either you are not eating enough of the nutrient-rich, energy-enhancing, healthy foods discussed earlier, or you are eating both, and therefore are consuming too many calories, which will cause you to end up overweight. Overweight in itself is an energy robber. Carrying more than a few pounds of surplus fat, if you don't already know, exhausting.

The Energy Robbers

Caffeine. Although thought of as a "pick-me-up" and a stimulant, caffeine unfortunately also appears to produce its own "low" after the "high" for many people. In other words if you use coffee, tea, chocolate, cola, or other caffeine-containing foods and drinks to boost your energy, you might suffer a rebound effect and feel worse than before. More caffeine will only establish a cycle of highs and lows. And for those sensitive to it, caffeine in excess of two or three cups of coffee can cause headaches, stomach aches, heartbeat irregularities, and insomnia. All of which will certainly rob you of energy.

Where to find the energy boosters

Beta-carotene
orange, yellow, and dark green vegetables, especially carrots, sweet potatoes pumpkin and squash tomatoes spinach broccoli watercress corn orange fruits, such as cantaloupe mangoes apricots peaches

Vitamin B^1 (*thiamine*)
sunflower and other sprouting seeds brown rice whole-grain cereals yeast extract wheat germ beans Brazil and other nuts

Vitamin B^2 (*riboflavin*)
yeast extract almonds and other nuts wheat germ cheese mushrooms broccoli yogurt beans eggs

Vitamin B^3 (*niacin*)
yeast extract beans whole wheat brown rice barley eggs meat fish

Vitamin B^6 (*pyridoxine*)
wheat germ soy oats walnuts and other nuts beans bananas avocados whole grains meat fish green vegetables sweet potatoes

Vitamin B^{12}
egg yolks cheese yeast extract milk fortified soy milk, seaweed

Vitamin C (*ascorbic acid*)
red peppers and chilies black currants parsley oranges and all other fresh fruit and vegetables *(Heat and light destroy vitamin C so fruits and vegetables must be stored in cool, dark conditions and eaten as soon after purchase as possible; eat raw or lightly cooked.)*

Vitamin E (*tocopherol*)
sunflower and other pure vegetable oils nuts seeds sweet potatoes avocados asparagus green vegetables barley soy beans brown rice

Iron
meat whole grains nuts eggs dark leafy greens beans seeds wheat germ dried apricots and peaches

Magnesium
all vegetables, especially green nuts seeds beans meat seafood figs bananas brown rice

Zinc
meat whole grains seafood eggs nuts beans

Selenium
liver kidneys lean meat seafood whole grains

Chemicals in food. Some believe that pesticides and other chemicals used in the mass production of food deplete or destroy the vital elements in the earth, such as magnesium and selenium. Chemicals and antibiotic residues also remain in and on produce, meat, and dairy products. Though there is much controversy as to their effect in the body, I strongly recommend not ingesting these substances. Whenever possible, choose organic foods grown or produced by people you know (grown by you is even better).

Allergens. Approximately one in ten people suffer from some form of food allergy. A wide variety of foods can produce allergic reactions, but the most common ones are wheat-based products, dairy products (particularly cow's milk and cheese), citrus fruits, certain nuts, and eggs. Food allergies can cause stomach bloating, lethargy, skin problems, and headaches. If you think you may have an allergy, it is wise to see a doctor who can arrange testing. If you want to self-test, cut out one food at a time from your diet for a period of two weeks each; if your symptoms disappear you may be allergic to that food. If on eating the food again the symptoms reappear, you are probably allergic to it.

Crash dieting. Most crash diets are woefully short in most of the nutrients essential to good health. Crash diets also cause fatigue and loss of lean body tissue (muscle), essential for a healthy metabolic rate, strength, and energy.

Two other factors can affect your body's ability to absorb the nutrients you need for energy:

Smoking
Depletes vitamin C and creates the need for extra antioxidants.

Stress
Depletes several vitamins and minerals, particularly the vitamin B group, vitamin C, magnesium, and zinc. This may be one reason why, when under stress, we are more susceptible to minor ailments.

And It's Not Just *What* You Eat . . .
How and when you eat can affect your energy levels almost as much as what you eat, so here are some guidelines to help you plan your meals to maximize vitality and minimize sluggishness.

• Avoid large meals. Your body has trouble digesting large amounts of food; to cope, blood is diverted from the brain, leaving you feeling fatigued or even sleepy, and causing your mental abilities to be temporarily impaired.

• Eat little and often. If you want to feel alert all day, eat several smaller meals evenly spaced throughout the day. Two medium-size meals (lunch and dinner), one small meal (breakfast), and two snacks (mid-morning and mid-afternoon) are ideal. All meals and snacks should contain some carbohydrates, some protein, and a small amount of fat for optimum blood sugar level control.

• Early in the day, you may want to avoid large portions of complex carbohydrates like breads, pasta, potatoes, or rice. "Heavy" carbohydrates like these have a mild sedative effect when eaten in large quantities. While most foods contain some carbohydrates, the simple carbohydrates of fruits, vegetables, and dairy products function as quick energy boosters. When combined with a small portion of complex carbs, you'll have a steady supply of energy all day. But if you want a "relaxing" meal at the end of the day, make your entrée a pasta or rice dish.

• Don't skip breakfast. You need its nutrients, especially its calories, for energy after the long night's fast. Without breakfast your blood sugar level will be low and you won't have the energy you need to get through the morning.

• Don't go hungry. The golden rule of eating for energy is, if you feel real hunger, eat a healthy snack, or set your eating timetable around your most hungry times.

• If you exercise (which you should be doing throughout the 10-week program and beyond), you need to bear a few nutrition points in mind to avoid muscle fatigue during exercise and muscle pain afterwards. Sports nutritionists often recommend eating a high carbohydrate snack an hour before exercising and drinking plenty of fluids before and during exercise. After exercising, eat a small carbohydrate snack and drink more fluids. Ideal carb snacks are dried apricots and figs, fresh bananas, yogurt, and rye crispbread with an apple and a small slice of reduced-fat cheese. The complex carbs—bread, pasta, potatoes, rice, cereal, or other grains are fine in moderation—either an hour before or soon after exercise, and are best eaten in combination with protein and a small amount of fat.

THE ZEST PLAN

If your diet has been particularly poor recently, with a lot of the energy robbers, consider this two-day Superhealth diet to give your body what it needs. Follow it for the two days, then move on to the Seven-Day Zest Plan.

Superhealth Diet
This is simplicity itself. Over two days eat and drink as much as you like (within reason–don't overdose on any one item) of the items listed below, plus the evening extras and a daily Energy Drink. The only rules are to eat when you are hungry, eat small amounts, and eat often. Also make sure you drink around two quarts of noncaffeinated fluid a day.

Eat or drink what you want of:
- Bottled noncarbonated mineral water
- Fresh fruit and raw vegetables
- Fresh fruit and vegetable juices
- Uncooked nuts (unsalted)
- Seeds
- Yogurt

Have one Energy Drink each morning:

Blend together
1 cup (250 ml) soy milk or skim milk
4½ ounces (125 g) fresh chopped fruit (for example, pineapple, raspberries, oranges)
1 small banana
3 tablespoons yogurt
1 teaspoon honey
1 teaspoon wheat-germ oil

In the evening on both days have 1 small baked potato in addition to any of the unlimited items above.

Seven-Day Zest Plan
The Seven-Day Zest Plan is based around those five-star energy foods and the when-and-how-to-eat guidelines covered in this workshop. Eating this way should have you feeling satisfied and replete, but also light, energetic, bright, and without uneven energy levels.

Tips
- *Eat organic foods whenever possible.*
- *Eat food in season when it is freshest and best.*
- *Cook vegetables or fruit minimally, if at all.*
- *Eat freely of the Unlimited Foods listed in the Size-wise Eating Plan on page 26.(Portion sizes aren't stated – eat only enough to satisfy your appetite and no more.)*
- *Never eat to the point of feeling full and/or sluggish.*
- *Eat slowly and chew thoroughly.*

BREAKFAST every day
Either one Energy Drink (see left) or portion of yogurt with chopped dried apricots or peaches, sunflower seeds, and a few rolled oats; plus 1 portion fresh fruit or portion yogurt with fruit compote (made by simmering a selection of dried fruits, including apricots, prunes, and apples, in orange juice until tender), topped with sunflower seeds and oats. Add some chopped fresh fruit before serving.

Two SNACKS every day
Choose two from this list (more if exercising, see opposite page):
- 2 rice cakes
- 1 portion citrus fruit
- 2 rye crispbreads with a little goat's cheese and 1 small apple
- Handful of homemade granola (containing plenty of nuts, seeds, and dried fruit) with a little skim milk
- Small banana and yogurt
- Handful of almonds or Brazil nuts and 1 peach or nectarine

- Handful of dried apricots or peaches with a tablespoon of sunflower seeds

FRESH FRUIT
When fruit is mentioned but not specified within the diet choose any fresh raw fruit but aim to eat plenty of: apricots, peaches, nectarines, melons, citrus fruits, berries, and pineapples.

LUNCH AND DINNER
DAY 1
Lunch Salad of blanched almonds, dried apricots, ripe avocado, and mixed greens (including a minimum of one dark leaf, such as spinach or watercress), all tossed in olive oil and lemon dressing; served with a small amount of rye bread.
Evening Casserole of diced chicken or tofu chunks with mushrooms, red bell peppers, and vegetable stock, and thickened with tomato paste. Serve with chopped green vegetables stir-fried very lightly in sunflower oil; baked sweet potato; fresh fruit.

DAY 2
Lunch Crab salad (dressed crab with slices of cantaloupe, chopped fresh herbs, and salad leaves) and rye crispbreads, followed by a selection of dried fruits and yogurt.
Evening Grilled, broiled, or baked trout or salmon with fresh peas or snow peas, broccoli, and potatoes, followed by fresh fruit.

DAY 3
Lunch Homemade carrot soup made by simmering and puréeing fresh chopped carrots with vegetable stock and tomatoes, seasoned with fresh coriander and sesame seeds, and swirled with yogurt; serve with small amount of rye bread and follow with fresh fruit.
Evening Tofu and mixed nuts stir-fried with bean sprouts, green

beans, snow peas, red bell peppers, and broccoli, lightly stirred in sunflower oil; served with brown rice or other whole grain.

DAY 4
Lunch Salad of goat's cheese, tomato, red onion, chopped garlic, and mixed greens, tossed in olive oil and lemon dressing; serve with whole-wheat pita bread and follow with fresh fruit.
Evening Homemade vegetable chili using chopped red chilies, selection of fresh vegetables, and canned beans of choice (pinto beans, lentils, chickpeas), simmered in a base of chopped tomatoes, vegetable stock, and onion; serve on grain of choice (buckwheat, barley, millet); mixed salad.

DAY 5
Lunch Homemade Lentil and Vegetable Soup (see page 32); wholewheat pita bread; fresh fruit.
Evening Spanish omelet filled with cooked potato, red bell peppers, peas, and parsley; mixed salad.

DAY 6
Lunch Salad of cooled cooked brown rice mixed with pine nuts, sunflower seeds, banana, and cantaloupe, plus a little chopped grilled chicken; fresh fruit to follow.
Evening Vegetarian pasta bake using whole-wheat pasta, cooked brown lentils, chopped nuts, chickpeas, and eggplant, with a fresh tomato sauce base and topped with a little grated cheese; serve with spinach, broccoli, and a sweet potato.

DAY 7
Lunch Salad of hard-boiled egg, tuna fish, red bell peppers, parsley, watercress, and salad greens of choice, tossed with olive oil and vinegar dressing; fresh fruit to follow.
Evening Classic bouillabaisse (fish stew) served with rye bread and mixed salad.

YOUR LONG-TERM DIET

You may repeat the Seven-Day Zest Plan for another week or two, but eventually you will want to devise your own diet. Use the following lists of high-energy foods to plan a well-balanced diet.

Five-Star Foods

These are foods that you should choose as often as you can because nutritionally they offer great value. As an example, white potatoes and sweet potatoes are similar in their content of calories, vitamin C, and fiber, and both are healthy, complex carbohydrate foods. But sweet potatoes are richer in more of the important nutrients, such as beta-carotene, than white potatoes, so they are on the five-star list, while white potatoes are on the three-star list.

Fresh Fruits: all, but particularly citrus fruits, avocados, apricots, peaches, nectarines, melons, berries, figs, mangoes, papaya, kiwi.

Dried fruits: apricots, peaches.

Vegetables: all green leafy vegetables and herbs; all orange, red, dark green vegetables; onions, garlic, corn.

Nuts and seeds: almonds, walnuts, sprouting seeds, sunflower seeds, sesame seeds.

Legumes: beans, lentils, chickpeas, split peas.

Grains: all whole grains, especially barley, buckwheat, millet, oats, rice, wild rice, rye.

Others: yogurt, oily fish, tofu, sunflower oil, linseed oil, rapeseed oil, olive oil.

Three-Star Foods

These are foods you can add to your five-star diet to provide variety and extra nutrients and calories.

Dried fruits: prunes, apples, figs, pears, raisins, currants.

Vegetables: potatoes, yams (white-fleshed), parsnips, artichokes, fresh beans, eggplants.

Nuts and seeds: all other nuts and seeds.

Grains and pasta: preferably whole-wheat, noodles, white rice, rye crispbreads, fortified white breads, rice cakes.

Others: eggs, lean meat and poultry, shellfish, liver, kidneys (unless pregnant), cheeses (in limited quantities), skim milk, unsalted butter (in limited quantity), spices, tomato paste.

Other Foods

These are foods you don't actually need to remain healthy but may find yourself wanting now and again. The longer you continue eating the Zest Plan way, though, the less you will have a taste for such foods. If you consume the following foods on occasion—and always in moderation—you will be fine, but if you consume more of these foods than of the five and three star fuel foods above, you will find your energy level and general health slipping again. *So beware!*

- All highly processed foods
- All foods high in saturated fat and/or sugar and low in nutrients (most cookies, candies, pastries, cakes, potato and corn chips)
- Condiments, such as mayonnaise and salt

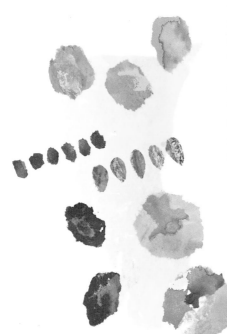

P hysical and mental stamina are faculties we tend to lose gradually as we age. Yet this "slowing down" isn't inevitable. With the right type of exercise–for both brain and body–you can recover the capabilities you had 10, even 20, years ago.

WORKSHOP 14   IMPROVE YOUR STAMINA

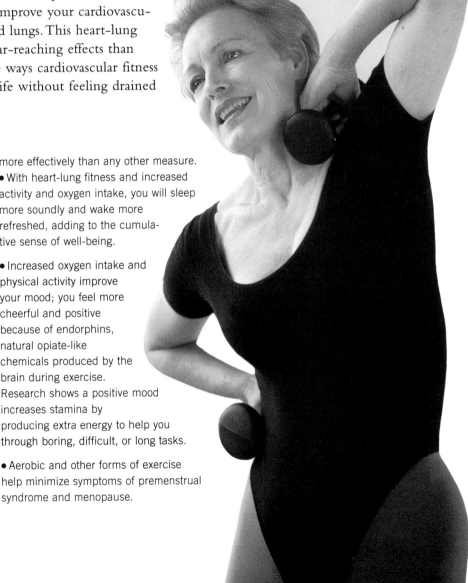

S leep, relaxation, a healthy diet, and fun in your life can all help your stamina levels. But the single most important factor is to "exercise for energy." You need to improve your cardiovascular fitness, the fitness of your heart and lungs. This heart-lung fitness–or lack of it–has much more far-reaching effects than you may realize. Here are some of the ways cardiovascular fitness can help you sail through your daily life without feeling drained or exhausted.

● A fit body is better able to cope with all the demands made on it, therefore it doesn't tire as quickly and can do more, work harder, and work longer.

● Your circulation, which is directly linked to the fitness of your heart and lungs, improves with exercise, increasing your metabolic rate. Everything is working faster and you feel more alert and more energetic. It also means, by the way, that you can turn down the central heating because you will naturally keep warmer–and an overheated room can be a major cause of lethargy.

● Oxygen intake improves as your heart fitness and lung capacity improve. As more oxygen and glucose reach the brain, your mental abilities increase, including concentration, memory, and reaction time. Research shows that physical exercise helps stop mental decline more effectively than any other measure.

● With heart-lung fitness and increased activity and oxygen intake, you will sleep more soundly and wake more refreshed, adding to the cumulative sense of well-being.

● Increased oxygen intake and physical activity improve your mood; you feel more cheerful and positive because of endorphins, natural opiate-like chemicals produced by the brain during exercise. Research shows a positive mood increases stamina by producing extra energy to help you through boring, difficult, or long tasks.

● Aerobic and other forms of exercise help minimize symptoms of premenstrual syndrome and menopause.

So how do you achieve cardiovascular fitness, especially if you've not raised a sweat for years? Any one of any age–as long as you have been given the okay by a physician–can improve cardiovascular fitness to the extent that you can turn back time. A sedentary person can increase aerobic capacity by up to 80 percent within 10 weeks of beginning a stamina-building program.

All you need to do is regular aerobic exercise suited to your own level of fitness. Aerobic exercise is any exercise sustained for at least 20 minutes that raises your pulse (gets your heart beating faster) and causes your lungs to work harder by taking in more oxygen.

And it really is never too late to start.

Making Your Body Work for You

The alternative–to continue "slowing down" and do no aerobic exercise at all–will condemn your body to unnecessary deterioration.

Before you begin an aerobic exercise program you must check that you don't have any contraindications. If you answer yes to any of the following questions, you *must* check with your physician before beginning the program that follows–or any other exercise program.

• **Are you age 50 or over and have done no formal exercise within the last five years?**
• **Do you have a Body Mass Index of 30 or more (see Workshop 1)?**
• **Are you suffering from any medical condition now, or have you recently?**

• **Are you pregnant or have you given birth within the past six weeks?**
• **Have you any physical condition that might make exercise difficult, such as back pain or arthritis?**

If you answered yes to any, see your doctor and show him or her this plan. Get an okay. Any of the above contraindications won't necessarily stop you from exercising, but your doctor will probably reassure you by checking blood pressure, heart rate, and so on.

Once you have the all-clear to exercise, you can proceed to the next test, which involves finding out how fit–or unfit–you are. For this, all you need to do is walk a measured mile.

The Measured Mile

• Measure a mile (1.6 km) walking route on flat, even ground, using a pedometer or a car (or measure it on a map as a last resort).
• Put on comfortable, cushioned walking shoes and comfortable clothes. Warm up by marching in place slowly for two minutes. Make sure you have a watch with a second hand.
• Start walking the mile route at as brisk a pace as you can manage without having to stop to get your breath back and while still being able to talk. If you are walking alone, count to 10 occasionally out loud, instead of talking.

You should feel your heart beating more strongly and be aware of your lungs working harder to take in more air than normal, but you shouldn't feel real discomfort, such as pain in your chest or lungs, or any burning in your leg muscles. If you do – stop, and start again, if you feel able, at a slower pace. If you can't complete the mile without discomfort–just stop and record how long you did walk.
• At the end of your mile, take note of how long it took you to cover it, and check it against the fitness level chart below.

Aerobics enhances your looks, too!

As a bonus, you will find aerobic exercise will help you look more youthful, too. The extra blood-flow to the skin (through better circulation) will improve your skin's condition, tightening pores, lessening pallor, and giving the skin a healthy glow. Even better, because aerobic exercise burns up calories, it helps you to get, or stay, slim.

Your Fitness Level

	35 or under	36–55	56+	
Couldn't walk the mile	A	B	C	A = *Extremely unfit*
Took over 20 minutes	B	C	D	B = *Very unfit*
Took 18–20 minutes	C	D	E	C = *Moderately unfit*
Took 15–17 minutes	D	E	F	D = *Slightly fit*
Took 14 minutes or less	E	F	G	E = *Fit*
Took 13 minutes or less	F	G	G+	F = *Very fit*
Took 12 minutes or less	G	G+	G++	G = *Superfit*

Your Fitness Program

Your main activity during the 10-week program will be to build up your stamina through walking. Walking is a good way to start a fitness regime because it is simple, cost-effective, can be done from your own home, requires little special equipment, and progress is easy to monitor.

All you have to do is go out and walk three times a week (four, if you like, in later weeks) and work through the fitness levels, opposite. For instance, if you are age 45 and you scored D on the fitness assessment, your goal is to reach G over the weeks ahead. If you are age 56 and you scored C on the fitness assessment, your goal is to reach F or better. Anyone–yes, anyone–can improve at least three levels during the 10-week program. Most of you will be able to improve right up to G.

Follow the instructions given for the Measured Mile, and gradually your times will improve. As your times improve, you will be getting fitter.

Here are some additional notes before you begin:

• If you already rate an F or G, you are already fit and need only maintain your current level of fitness for adequate stamina. This will entail walking at level F or G three times a week for 20 minutes or more (obviously you will be walking more than a mile in this case). If you want to increase your fitness level, you will need to work your body harder, which will mean something such as hill-walking, jogging (only advisable in top-quality shoes, on an unpaved surface, and if you have no joint problems), circuit training in the gym, or cycling.

• Every time you walk, don't forget that to increase fitness you must raise your heart rate and feel your lungs working. Work as hard as you can within the "talk test" level. As long as you keep doing that, you will keep improving.

• Walk with good form–upright with tummy and bottom tucked in, legs striding out from hips, shoulders relaxed and down, eyes looking forward (not down), arms swinging naturally by sides.

• Don't forget a two-minute warm-up, and it is a good idea to have a two-minute cool-down, too (the leg stretches on page 37 are also a good thing).

• Once you've worked up to level F or G, you should continue walking after the measured mile to complete a minimum of 20 minutes. If you walk longer than that, you will get fitter more quickly and you will burn extra calories, so don't think of the 20 minutes as a maximum–it's a minimum.

• Most people will be able to progress one level per three to six sessions (one to two weeks). Make this your goal.

What to Do When You Can't Walk

What do you do if the weather is too bad to walk or it's too dark out there? Consider other aerobic options. If your walk really is off today, it is better to do something rather than nothing.

Here are some first-choice options:

• Invest in an indoor aerobic machine. The cross-country ski machine is low-impact (easy on your joints), exercises all your major muscles at once, is quiet and is fun to use. During the winter months I can't remember how I used to get by without it. Other choices are an exercise cycle, a rower, or a treadmill.

• Buy a step. It gives a good lower body and cardiovascular workout like walking and cycling and burns about the same number of calories. You'll need a video to go with it, otherwise it gets boring.

• Buy an aerobics video. There are plenty of good ones for sale–all you need is a reasonable space in front of the TV. Some have routines that are quite difficult to follow at first, something to beware of if you have two left feet.

• Buy a mini-trampoline (rebounder). It's good for low-impact exercise, and ideal for people with joint problems.

Second-choice options:

• Buy a jump rope. This is fabulous aerobic exercise but if you are unfit it is very difficult to keep up for longer than a minute or two. Also, you need to do it outdoors or in a high-ceilinged room. However, if you do persist, your minute session will soon progress to five minutes, and five minutes of skipping is very good cardiovascular exercise.

• Stairs. If you have stairs, climb up them at a pace to get your heart rate raised and your lungs working. Keep it up for several minutes.

• Marching/jogging in place. If all else fails, march vigorously in place for several minutes. Start off at a warm-up pace, then gradually get faster, raising knees higher and pumping arms harder. When you finish, slow down to cool down.

MIND GAMES

Your brain power will improve as your physical stamina improves, but you can do still more to give your mind back its sharp edge.

Try these ideas:

Give yourself air. Your brain needs fresh air so never waste an opportunity to give it some.

Mental exercises. Improve your brain's stamina through the mental equivalent of aerobic exercises. For concentration–turn a book or newspaper upside down and continue reading for as long as you can. Time yourself. Do it longer tomorrow. For memory–read a small paragraph in a book or newspaper once, put it away, and try to memorize it. Tomorrow, try to do better. Once you can do one paragraph, make it two. For sharpness–time yourself while you go through the alphabet out loud attaching a word to each letter. Tomorrow, do it quicker. Then do two words to each letter, then three.

Stretch your mind at every opportunity; instead of buying a steamy best-seller for a trip, get a novel that will make you think more.

Do something different. If you are set in many habits, alter as many as you can. If you always follow the same pattern when you get up, change it. If you always read the paper in a certain order, alter it. If you always go to the same supermarket and shop in the same order, go somewhere else. If your mind is fed the same diet, it loses its powers of enquiry and observation.

Supplement? Gingkho Biloba and L-Carnitine are two supplements said to improve mind stamina and energy. Taken as instructed they should have no side effects so you may want to give them a try.

*H*ow long has it been since you really relaxed? One of the largest drains on energy is a state of near-permanent stress. Yet for very many women, that is how they live their lives.

 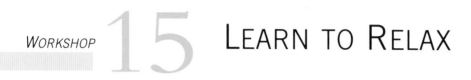

15 LEARN TO RELAX

The more time you spend not relaxing, the harder it is to do. And, the more it shows in your appearance. A recent major study showed that women subject to a period of anxiety began to look older within months–but if they could learn to relax and minimize stress, they began to look younger again. This workshop is concerned with teaching you to wind down and letting your body and mind recharge their energy levels.

Relax Your Body

These are symptoms indicating you need to relax your body:

- Frequent headaches
- Difficulty sleeping
- Heartburn
- Fast pulse without exertion
- Difficulty in taking a deep breath
- Shallow breathing
- Voice high, hoarse
- Area where skull meets neck sore when gently pressed

- Shoulders up high, knotted muscles easily felt on each side of neck
- Teeth clenched, jaw stiff
- Physical nervous habits: nail biting, hair twisting, nose scratching, fingernails digging into palms
- Toes bunched up inside shoes

How many of these symptoms is your body displaying now? The more you have, the less relaxed you are. These physical symptoms are symptoms of your unrelaxed mind and unrelaxed lifestyle. Like unraveling a ball of yarn, you need to teach your body to relax, then tackle the problems causing that tension.

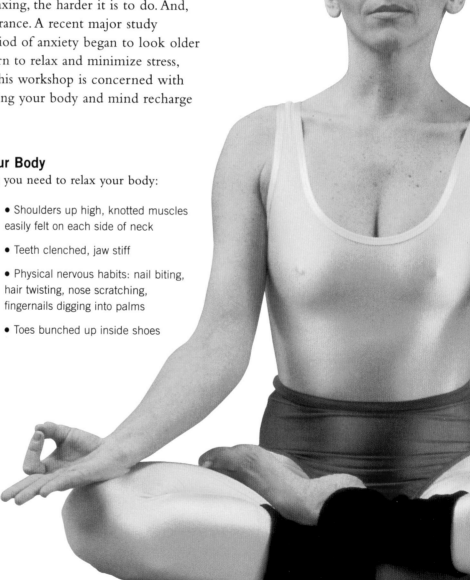

Through Exercise

As we saw in Workshop 14, exercise is a great giver of energy, turning a lethargic body and a slow mind into energized vital ones. But almost as importantly, it is a wonderful natural relaxant. If only every one who uses tranquilizers, sleeping pills, alcohol, or drugs in their attempts to relax would just try exercising first!

Exercise relaxes you in several ways. Aerobic exercise releases natural chemicals, called endorphins, that improve your mood. It also warms up your body—a similar effect to taking a "relaxing" hot bath. And it disperses a buildup of adrenaline common in people who are stressed out. Adrenaline builds up in response to stress as the body prepares to "fight or flight," but in modern life our fights are more likely to be verbal than physical, and we don't run away—so the adrenaline stays in our bodies causing increased blood pressure and heart rate, and muscle tension. As aerobic exercise mimics "fight or flight," it works perfectly to calm us down.

A period of exercise in a different environment—say, walking—gets you away from whatever is tensing you up and gives you time to cool off and calm down. Lastly, if you are tense, you hold your muscles taut, causing lactic acid to build up in them, resulting in aching and stiffness and making it difficult to relax the muscles

without help. Activity of the right kind—say, a stretching session—can release those muscles.

The 10-week program includes regular aerobic activity and a stretching session to finish your Total Tone routine three times a week. The Long Body Stretch (see page 51) is a wonderful tension releaser at any time, but if you score very high on the list of tension symptoms, opposite, you may want to build more relaxing exercises into your daily life. Here are some guidelines:

• Do your aerobic exercise at a time of day when you are most likely to be stressed—for example, if you wake in the morning feeling tense about the day ahead, take your walk then. If a bad day leaves you tense, the activity taken then will help you to relax through the evening. The 10-week program suggests aerobic exercise three times a week, but you can increase this (once you are fit enough to cope) to up to six times a week.

• On days you are not doing the Total Tone routine, do the Warm-up and Cool-down stretches one after the other, twice a day. This will take you about eight minutes a session. Once you are used to the stretches you can do them longer.

• Consider adding a yoga session into your schedule. Yoga relaxes the mind and the body at the same time and creates energy.

SIX INSTANT WAYS TO RELAX

❶ **Clench your jaw** by biting teeth together hard. Now open your mouth as wide as you can and say, "Aaaah!"

❷ **Sigh** as loudly and as deeply as you can, then take in a good breath of fresh air.

❸ **Smile.** Even better, laugh. Laughter is a physical and mental relaxer.

❹ **Do a few neck rolls.** Sit with spine upright and shoulders as relaxed as possible. Slowly let your head drop toward your right shoulder as far as it can go, return to the center and let it drop slowly to the left. Repeat 5 times.

❺ **Shrug your shoulders.** With arms at your sides, lift your shoulders up toward your ears as high as possible, then pull them down as far as possible. Repeat 5 times.

❻ **Face massage.** Starting in the center of your forehead, and using first and second fingers of both hands, gently make small circular motions (clockwise with your right fingers, counterclockwise with your left), gradually moving your fingers across your forehead to the temples then, even more gently, down beside your eyes and in across the cheekbones to your nose. Feel those tension lines around your eyes disappear!

The Benefits of Massage

For thousands of years the relaxing benefits of a good body massage have been appreciated.

Massage calms the nerve receptors in the skin, decreases blood pressure and pulse rate, promotes removal of lactic acid in the muscles, and induces deeper breathing and a sense of well-being.

I believe that even if a woman does not have the time or money for any other luxury or perk in her life, she should make the time and find the money, if necessary, for a regular massage session.

If you feel too guilty for such indulgence, perhaps Section Three—and particularly Workshop 24—will help you change your mind. However, even if you don't pick up the phone and book that massage, you can sample its benefits with the short self-massage explained below. Even better, if you have a partner you can try techniques out on each other.

It is also well worth learning the basics of reflexology—a form of massage relatively easy to carry out on yourself.

Self-massage

Work on your "trigger points"—those painful nodules caused by stress and which can lead to a muscle spasm, reduction of blood flow to the area, and build up of lactic acid. Using finger pressure on the trigger points you can disperse the lactic acid, get the blood flowing again, and therefore relax the muscle. Use finger pressure as firm as you can bear and hold for a slow count of 10 unless otherwise stated. Don't use massage oil.

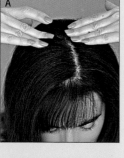

1. Use the third and fourth finger of each hand to press the crown of your head (photo A).

2. Using your thumb, press at 1-inch intervals along the base of the skull, f t one side and then the other (photo B).

3. Using left-hand fingers, squeeze right side of neck, then use right-hand fingers on left side of neck.

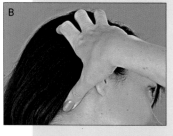

4. Use right-hand fingers to press the muscle at the back of the left shoulder in the triangle between the collarbone and the shoulder blade. You will immediately know when you have found the right spot! Repeat on the other side (photo C).

5. Move fingers slightly further in toward spine and press again. Repeat to other side.

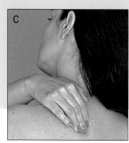

Reflexology

In reflexology, pressure is exerted with the fingers or thumbs on reflex points in the feet that some believe correspond to different parts of the body. The toes correspond to the head and neck. The farther down toward the heel of the foot the nearer you get to the lower body.

If your neck is tight, the inner side and base of your big toe will be very sore when pressed; if your shoulders are tense, the ball of your foot just below the little toe will be correspondingly sore. To work the spine, press all along the inside edge of each foot, from the big toe to the heel, following the line of the arch of the foot. But an all-over foot massage—five minutes each foot using firm pulsing finger or thumb pressure at ½ inch intervals—is very relaxing in itself. We don't give our feet enough attention and having them "worked over" is a real pleasure.

To do self-reflexology, sit on the floor or bed with legs crossed. Use the right hand to work the left foot and vice versa, and use the non-working hand to hold the foot firmly. Hold the heel if working the toe area and the toes if working the heel or middle foot. If you find a particularly tender area, give it extra time.

Breathing

If you are tense you are likely to be breathing very shallowly and too quickly, which means your body will not be getting enough oxygen—a symptom of which is, ironically, anxiety. Your lungs will not be expelling the waste—gases, carbon dioxide—efficiently, either, a symptom of which is fatigue. This self-perpetuating vicious circle needs to be broken if you are to feel better. Deep breathing can calm you down within minutes and will also energize you.

If possible, lie down wearing loose clothing. Exhale through the mouth, as long as you can. Inhale through the mouth, to a count of 10, feeling your diaphragm (under your ribcage) and your abdomen rise. Try to get in enough air to fill your lungs completely. Now slowly exhale to a count of 20, trying to push every last breath of air from those lungs. Try this for two or three minutes.

When you go about your normal routine, keep remembering to give yourself oxygen! Get rid of all that carbon dioxide! BREATHE!

Now Relax Your Mind

Many of us live with negative stimuli like these every day of our lives and don't realize what a huge impact they have on us. Some can perhaps be altered; others aren't so easy to do anything about. But what you need to do is find that block of time at least once a day to create your own positive, calming environment.

Increase positive calming influences

Create your own calming environment by using one or several of the following suggestions:

- Use blackout eye-mask and earplugs to counteract negative noise and sight stimuli.

- Use a personal audio instead of earplugs to listen to relaxing music or sounds you enjoy.

- Walk in a pretty and quiet place. Even in the middle of a city there are parks and gardens to enjoy.

- Make your own retreat. Create one place that is for you and you alone to relax in and enjoy. A corner of a room if not a whole room, a spot in the garden or, if you have nowhere else, make the bathroom your refuge. Inside your refuge always push anxious thoughts away and practice letting your mind float. Allow only good thoughts to intrude. Breathe deeply.

TRY A RETREAT

Why not try a week at a retreat this year for your vacation, or if you haven't that much time, a weekend? Retreats are geared to stress reduction, relaxation, peace, and healing. You will find exercise, massage, counseling, and more at most retreats and the cost is usually much less than that of health spas or resorts.

You need to relax your mind if:

- You skip from one chore to another without completing any.

- You can't concentrate on reading.

- You can't "switch off" your mind at the end of the day.

- You worry about trivial things that don't bother other people.

- It doesn't take much to make you lose your temper.

- People tell you things but they don't seem to stay in your brain.

There's a lot going on inside your head, but that's not necessarily a good thing! If you said "yes" to more than one item on the above list, it's time to calm down, clear your mind, and relax. You need to look at your lifestyle and reorganize it so you don't keep going into "overload" (Workshops 12 and 17 to 24 will help), but there are also plenty of immediate solutions.

At least once a day, you need to make time for yourself, during which you will learn the technique of mental relaxation.

Reduce negative stimuli

Here are some of the outside stimuli that may be adding to your mental tension:

- Loud, noisy music of a type you don't enjoy.

- People shouting or talking too loudly, especially about some thing you find distasteful or boring.

- Television on too loud.

- Traffic noise.

- Bright lights, particularly flashing.

- Insistent noise, such as a hammer hitting, or a road drill.

- More than one person trying to talk to you at the same time.

- Crowded space, such as in a train, or at a party.

- Phone ringing constantly.

- The essential aromatherapy oils ylang ylang, valerian, chamomile and lavender applied in firm stroking movements to your forehead and chest will calm you down. The homeopathic remedy arg nit. (argentum nitricum) is worth trying, too.

- Use color. Avoid rooms or clothes in red, purple, and orange. Blues and greens are the most soothing colors–another reason why a walk in the country is relaxing.

- Use food. A diet high in potassium and carbohydrates is a calming one. Eat extra bananas, bread, watercress, and celery.

Learn to focus

The unrelaxed mind is likely to be focusing on too many things at once. Learn techniques to help you focus on one thing at a time.

- Decide on paper, in what order you are going to tackle things and stick to the order. At first you may only be able to do the first two things on the list in a focused, orderly way without straying. However, if you keep focusing every day gradually you will improve.

- Use meditation. During your quiet time of day (see left), sit and relax as much as possible and breathe deeply. Focus your eyes on a point ahead of you. Clear your mind of everything. If a thought comes into your head, banish it (try putting it in an imaginary balloon and letting it float off above your head and out of the room). Think of a relaxing word and keep repeating it. Meditate for 5 minute or longer.

- Count down from 100. See how far you can get before an extraneous thought comes into your head. When it does, try the balloon trick, above, and start counting from 100 again. Eventually you should be able to get to zero without losing focus.

Long Term

To achieve a lasting relaxed frame of mind, you need to work on the major causes of your day-to-day tension. Your body and your mind are, after all, just reflecting what is going on in your life when they get overstressed and seize up, or go into overdrive.

Section Three, beginning on page 118, will help you decide what it is you really want and will give you some ideas on how to make changes. Some things, of course, you cannot change; at least not for the moment. If that is the case, then you should spend your daily "quiet time" planning for the future in a positive way. But don't be too hard on yourself; and don't expect miracles. You will never be able to relax if you always feel as though you are one step short of where you want to be. Perhaps where you are *now* is not such a bad place after all. Use your quiet time to ponder on *that* thought tomorrow.

A good night's sleep ... a simple, natural process; the end result of a busy and tiring day–or something you haven't experienced in ages and would kill for. This workshop discusses how to improve the quality of your sleep without resorting to drugs.

Sleep problems tend to fall into two categories: trouble getting to sleep when you go to bed, and waking after two or three hours and finding it impossible to get back to sleep. We look at both scenarios here. Review the ideas and pick the ones that most suit your situation.

WORKSHOP 16 DEEP SLEEP

DON'T . . .

Go to bed if you're not really tired. Stay out of the bedroom until you feel tired.

Sleep in the morning to make up for a bad night's sleep. This will disrupt your body clock and make it even more difficult to get a good night's sleep the next night. It is better to be a little tired for one day, get some outdoor exercise, and try all the ideas in this workshop to make sure you sleep well the next night. The odd bad night won't harm you.

Sleep longer than necessary. In the winter it may be a nice idea to cuddle up, turn over, and go back to sleep, but when you wake up naturally, it means you have had enough sleep. Too much sleep will leave you lethargic and more likely to have a restless night's sleep the next night.

Take sleeping pills except as a last resort. Natural sleep is what you need. And taken more than occasionally, sleeping pills gradually lose their effect, leaving you with few options, except to take stronger and stronger doses. In other words, they are addictive.

Regular, restful sleep is vital for a healthy and energized body and mind. Lack of sleep weakens the immune system and can lead to an increase in severity and number of illnesses; it can also affect concentration, memory, and creativity. Tiredness resulting from lack of sleep brings a host of its own problems, such as irritability and uneven emotional responses, and is linked with a high proportion of accidents.

A good night's sleep is also vital for maintaining a youthful appearance because, during sleep, growth hormones are released, renewing and repairing the tissues and cells of the body, including the skin. Even after one poor night's sleep, physical symptoms begin to show; dark circles and/or puffiness around the eyes, pale complexion. No wonder they call it "beauty sleep!"

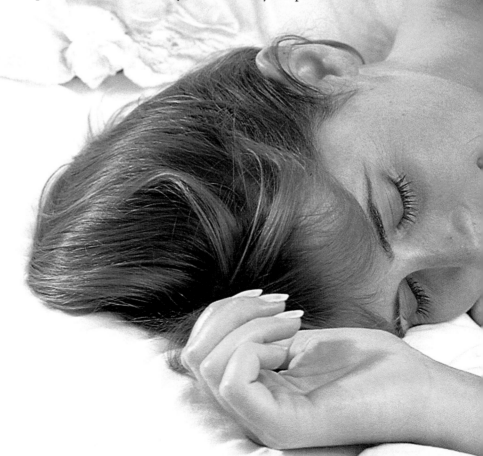

Getting to Sleep

During the day, make sure you engage in some at least one session of outdoor activity – the fresh air and the exercise will help you sleep. Your brain may be tired but your body needs to be tired, too, to sleep well. Follow a routine, when your work has finished, and which will gradually ready you for bed:

● Try to put the day's worries and problems behind you by making a "to do" list for the next day. Decide what you will wear tomorrow and get the outfit ready.

● Eat and drink to help you sleep. A small snack containing carbohydrates, calcium, and magnesium about one hour before bedtime will help calm your brain down. A cup of warm milk, a small banana, and a few crackers are ideal. Yogurt with chopped banana is another good idea. Such foods help the production of seratonin in your body–a neurotransmitter essential for good sleep. Don't eat or drink hard-to-digest foods late at night, such as cheese, red meat, or beans. If you like wine, one glass of red wine will act as a relaxant and help you to sleep, but more alcohol than that can severely disrupt your sleep later in the night. Avoid caffeine drinks such as coffee, tea, and cola, which are stimulants.

● If possible, follow a bath-stretch-and-massage routine before bed.

● Review your bedroom for sleep disturbers and sleep enhancers:

Avoid an overheated room. It is nice to go to bed in a warm room, but a stuffy atmosphere is one of the major causes of restlessness.

Avoid light. If you have to sleep in daylight, try blackout curtains or an eye mask. Don't leave electrical lights on.

Avoid noise. Your sense of hearing doesn't switch off when you are asleep and any loud, persistent, or sudden noise can wake you. Try to eliminate the causes of noise. Ask people not to bang doors shut, to turn music down, to talk more

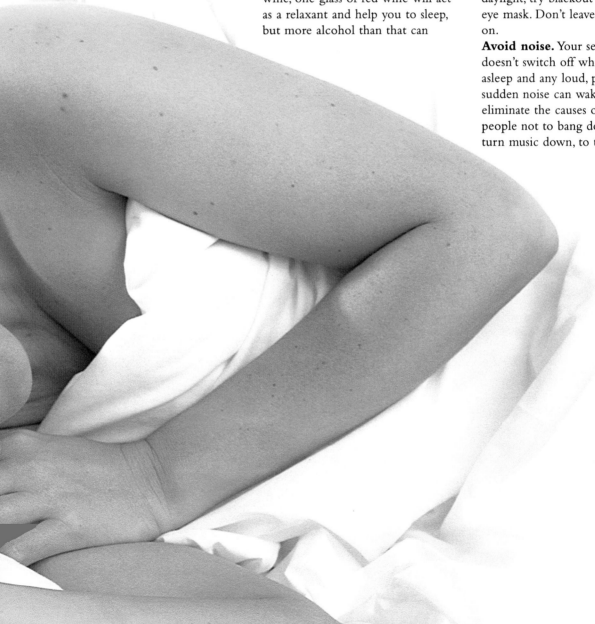

gently, and so on. If you can't eliminate the disturbances, wear earplugs.

Avoid an uncomfortable bed.
Sounds simple, but many people sleep on poor mattresses. You spend a third of your life on it, so get one you like. The same for pillows. A soft but supportive pillow is important; a hard, lumpy one can keep you awake.

Open the window. Fresh air circulating in the room is very important.

Decorate with calming, warm earth colors. Have things around you that make you feel secure–an old soft toy, furniture you like, an old duvet.

Enjoy an herbal tea just before sleeping. An infusion of 1 teaspoon dried, or 2 teaspoons fresh, herbs such as chamomile in ½ cup boiling water, left for 10 minutes and then strained is a good sleep inducer.

Go for natural remedies to control hormonal sleep disturbances. During menopause and in the week before a period, some women find they sleep poorly. This is due to hormonal disruption at these times. If this is your problem, try the essential oil clary sage in a bath or mixed with an almond oil base as a massage oil. Borage oil (starflower oil) is also good.

Go for good sex. Love-making promotes good sleep, so make time for an active sex life.

One or more of the above measures should be enough to send you to a restful sleep, but if you feel you need extra help, many people swear by several of the herbal sleep remedies on the market. My favorite is passionflower. But there are many others you can try, each with its own slightly different formula. The herbs used most often are valerian, chamomile, hops, and passionflower. It's really a matter of trial-and-error to see which works for you.

Waking in the night

Many people find they go to sleep perfectly well at bedtime but then wake a few hours later and lie there for two, three, or more hours unable to get back to sleep. This pattern will certainly be helped by the measures outlined on page 113 and left, but there are a few extra points worth mentioning:

● High alcohol intake is linked to poor sleep quality, particularly three to four hours after going to bed. So if you're drinking more to help you sleep–forget it. A cup of chamomile tea or other herbal sleeping aid or a small carbo-rich snack before bed are much more sensible alternatives.

● If you wake in the middle of the night at a similar time for more than a few nights in a row, it can become a habit the body adjusts to, and one difficult to break. Try going to bed later, or earlier, or sleeping in a different room for a night or two, to break this pattern.

● Waking in the early hours can be a sign of depression, in which case you should see your physician, or it can be unresolved anxieties or worry about a future event waking you up. If either of these last two is the case, you are likely to wake with a panicky feeling, perhaps with your heart racing. Try to use daytime hours to work through your worries and resolve them. Just talking to someone about them can be a great help. Fears always seem worse in the night when everyone else is asleep and it is dark. If this is your problem, take a cup of chamomile tea or other herbal aid when you wake, if it is more than four hours before you are due to get up. If it is only two or three hours before your normal waking time, a better course of action is to get up, move to a daytime room and do something pleasant such as reading, listening to music, or watching TV. In summer you can go out for an early walk. If it is work that is worrying

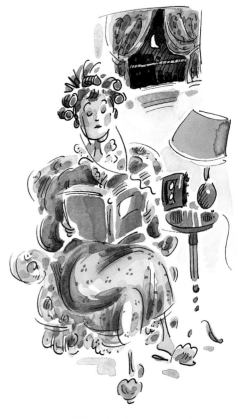

you, try tackling it–the positive feeling you get from doing something constructive about your problem is the first step toward breaking poor sleeping habits permanently.

● Shiftwork or jetlag could cause you to wake at odd hours. In that case try taking melatonin tablets to get you back on course. These are available over the counter in many outlets in the U.S. but not in Canada, but I wouldn't advise taking them on a permanent basis, because they still have to be thoroughly tested for long-term side effects. However, they seem to be better than sleeping pills.

● Bad dreams may wake you up in the last half of the night, because it is then that you have most rapid-eye-movement (REM) sleep, during which you dream. Some people find they have fewer disturbing dreams if they avoid caffeine, cheese, chocolate, and heavy meals in the evening. If you have many dreams that worry you, it would probably be a good idea to see a counselor.

*P*ositive thought is energy-giving and brings results. Negative thought is enervating and invites failure. It is also aging and unattractive. So take a lesson in zapping those negative feelings right out of your life.

WORKSHOP **17** # ZAPPING THE NEGATIVE

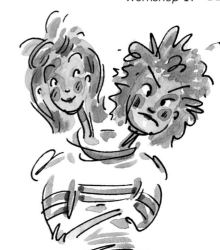

A r e   y o u   a   n e g a t i v e   p e r s o n   o r   a   p o s i t i v e   o n e ?

Answer the questions below to find out.

1 *You begin a new eating and fitness plan to get in shape but after a week you feel achy and hungry. Do you*

❑ *a.* Give up all idea of getting in shape but feel guilty about it?

❑ *b.* Accept it may have been the wrong plan for you and find a more gentle regimen that does suit you?

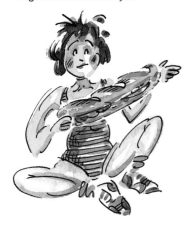

2 *Someone new moves in next to you. You take an instant dislike to her/him. Do you*

❑ *a.* Avoid her/him and begin house hunting?

❑ *b.* Make a deliberate effort to be friendly and pleasant, giving her/him the benefit of the doubt?

3 *You're passed over for a job at work because you are not experienced enough. The successful candidate arrives. Do you*

❑ *a.* Seethe inside every time you take an order from him/her and give up trying?

❑ *b.* Be gracious but twice as determined to get the job you want?

4 *Your ex-husband marries again. Are you more likely to*

❑ *a.* Find yourself bad mouthing his new wife at every opportunity and refusing to talk to her?

❑ *b.* Try to appear civil and pleased for them?

5 *You are on vacation with two days left. Which do you say?*

❑ *a.* Oh, dear, only two days to go; might as well start packing.

❑ *b.* Great! Two whole days left, let's see how much we can fit in!

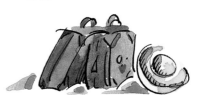

Yes, you know perfectly well A answers are negative and B answers are positive! Negative thoughts, words, feelings, and actions can eat up most of your day if you are not careful–and they can be very habit-forming.

There are two ways to tackle negativity:

1 Act or think positive even if you don't feel it inside. The right feelings often follow.

2 Understand the reasons for your negativity and overcome them.

Let's look at these two points as they apply to the types of negativity we experience most often.

Guilt–the Woman's Backpack

Most women are burdened with feelings of guilt to some degree. However much you do in your working day, however hard you try to see your friends and look after your family, however many meals you cook or cakes you bake, your efforts never quite seem good enough–so you feel guilty. I know friends who are wracked with guilt for not giving their cat enough attention or because they gave their sons the same sandwiches five days in a row for school lunch.

Take this to its logical conclusion and you could literally feel guilty about every single decision you make in the day. You only put 50 cents in the charity box–guilty! You ate two chocolate cookies–guilty! You cut short your telephone conversation with your mother, you should have found a better card for your friend's birthday, you only got through half your report revision, you weren't pleasant enough to the teller in the bank . . .

Really ridiculous, isn't it? You must begin to think positively. Practice turning every negative, guilty feeling and thought into one of pride in yourself. Try it with the situations above:

- I am a cat lover. I have a happy, healthy, well-fed cat who gets more attention than most cats I know.
- I make my son a wholesome packed lunch every day rather than letting him buy junk food like some of his friends. Ham is one of his favorite sandwiches.

- I put some money in a charity box today. It wasn't one of my favorite charities, but I like to help people when I can.
- I felt like treating myself so I ate two chocolate chip cookies–wasn't I good? I could have eaten the whole box!
- I call my mother most days and talk with her as long as I can even when I am busy.
- I remembered my friend's birthday and sent her a card even though she forgot mine last time.
- My revision was a lot harder than I had anticipated–but even so, I managed half of it.
- I had to wait 10 minutes in line and nearly missed my train, but I managed not to take it out on the teller.

Notice that the positive thoughts are more validating of yourself than the guilt feelings. Take an objective view of what you do and you will find you have little cause to feel guilty. If you do have valid cause to feel guilty, for example, if you beat the kids, keep your elderly mother locked up in an attic, starve the cat, or habitually rob banks, then you need to alter your behavior before you can alter your guilt. Ironically, however, truly wicked people rarely feel guilty.

If you aren't the type that feels guilty about everything but have strong guilt feelings about one particular area of your life–say, you can't see your elderly parents often because you live too far away–consider altering your circumstances to take away

the guilt. But look at the pros and cons of such decisions carefully. For instance, if you move to be near them, will you then feel guilty because you are far from your grandchildren? When you have to make a decision based on a best compromise, stick with it and use positive thoughts to feel good about the decision you have made.

Why, then, do you allow so many guilt feelings to ruin your confidence and sap your energy? Guilt without a real cause is pointless. Look back and see if you can find the answers. They could go back to your childhood and later years: how your parents treated you, how lovers treated you. If you discover you haven't been appreciated enough, you most likely have been trying to be perfect so you can be loved. To delve into such feelings you might want to consider counseling. But you don't necessarily need counseling to find the cure.

Keep turning those negative guilty thoughts into positive ones, and gradually you will feel more confidence and more pride in yourself and your achievements. You will come to appreciate yourself. And that is an important lesson to learn.

Handling Anger

Anger is not necessarily a negative emotion–it can be useful to kick-start you into doing something that needs doing (writing to the county government to complain about a dangerous road, for example). But if you feel intense anger a lot of the time you need to examine the cause(s) and deal with them. Women are usually bad at expressing anger and good at repressing it. Expressed anger is negative for the people on the receiving end; repressed anger is negative for you–it's bad for your health and zaps your energy.

Write a letter to yourself explaining what is making you angry. Many women feel anger because they feel used or abused, taken for granted, or helpless in a situation. Many charitable or local agencies can offer assistance or advice on where to seek help.

Envy–the "Eat You Up" Emotion

Envy–and its relatives, bitterness and resentment–are the most negative of all emotions. You want what someone else has–a good job, wealth, a particular house, a painting, a talent, a man, a physical attribute, a certain personality, an ability to attract friends . . .

If you find yourself envying somebody because of anything they are or have, remember this two-point plan.

First, think positively by using what I call the "trade-off" technique. Instead of thinking of the thing you want, focus on the things he or she might envy *you* for. Think of something you have that you wouldn't want to change, for example, "I really covet her long legs but I wouldn't swap my eyes or my hair." Focus on all the positive things in your life. If you do it often enough your envy will diminish. You can't be a copy of someone else – and if you could, you wouldn't want to be.

Second, understand that a common cause of envy is that you aren't investing enough time, thought, and planning into making your own life work. So stop envying – start planning. Start with strategies for banishing boredom, for improving your looks (well, you're doing that already with this program), for getting the career, for learning the talent, or whatever it is you envy in others. There may be some things beyond your limits for now, but there will be plenty you can do. Use Workshops 18 to 24 to help you.

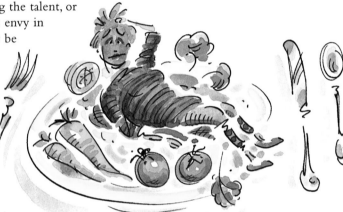

You can use these same techniques to help banish another emotion similar to envy–a general feeling of dissatisfaction with your life, your surroundings, your lot. In this instance, you haven't focused your dissatisfaction on someone else, but the negative emotion is still the same. Think of the positive sides of your life and take action to improve the rest.

Facing your Fears

As we get older, we feel we have more to lose. We get to appreciate the familiar things and begin to fear some of the rest. It's no wonder we feel fear. A little fear for the future is a good thing because it makes you appreciate what you have now. But when fear overtakes you and stops you from enjoying the moment or from making changes, it needs taming. This three-point plan will work.
On a piece of paper, divide your fears into three categories:
1 Fears that may never happen (something dreadful happening to one of your children, your partner leaving you).
2 Fears that will definitely or almost definitely happen (your children will grow up and leave home).
3 Fears connected with your lack of self-confidence (how will you get through that retraining

program, that speech you have to deliver).
Now make the positive thoughts for each fear. Here are examples:
"I am doing everything I can within reason to prevent anything awful happening to my children."
"I have a good relationship with my children. We can call or visit and I'll have more time for my hobbies."
"I have been accepted in this course/asked to make this speech, therefore I can do it."
Now try to understand why you have these fears.
For instance, if you have a lot of fears in group one – fears that may never come true – you need to tackle the reasons for that. You may need counseling to help you see the future as something good and exciting, rather than bleak and worrying.
If you have a lot of fears in

group two the best cure is to make certain you are doing everything in your power to make the most of the people, the places, the times that you value now. Make sure you give love and thought and time and appreciation and take what is offered gladly. Grabbing the moment now is an action you can take – and action beats fear.
If you have a lot of fears in group three you need to strengthen your self-esteem. This will come through doing what it is you fear. The more you turn away from things you fear the harder it gets to face them next time, the smaller your world becomes, and the lower your self-esteem.

Last Word . . .

There are, of course, plenty of other negative emotions that can sap your energy and upset your life. If you find yourself being negative in any situation, use the two-point method to get back to a positive frame of mind. Remember, positive-thinking is an energy source, and energy leads to a fulfilling life. Conversely, a fulfilling life can also give you energy. The next section, Life Choices–The Inner You, examines all the ways you can make your own life more fulfilling.

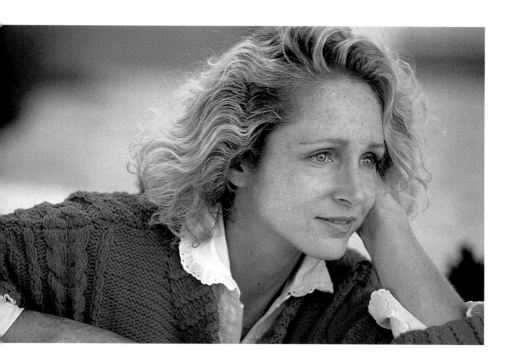

LIFE CHOICES

The Inner You

This section is all about the possibilities in your life. Find out what they are, decide which of them you really want, and turn them into reality. One of the most important differences between youth and old age is that young people dream, plan, plot, "go for it"—and if something doesn't work out, then they move on to something new without too much regret. At least they tried! Older people, however, don't do this. Or, at least, the older we get the less inclined we are to do so. We tend to put on blinkers, and life's possibilities narrow because of them. Attitudes harden, dreams get forgotten. But it doesn't need to be like that.

In our middle years, we can stay young in spirit if we hold onto that youthful mobility of thought, and by never letting a year of life go by without taking stock and planning new goals. It's not just new goals and adventures you need in life; you also need to look at the familiar to see how you can improve your quality of life, too. In this section you will learn to do all you can to revive your enthusiasm, restore your confidence and zest for life, and reevaluate your position, your values, your needs, and your relationships.

*W*hether you're bored with your job and want a complete change or just feel it's time for a promotion, or if you haven't worked for years and want a new start but feel out of touch, here's how to revamp your career potential for the 21st century.

WORKSHOP 18 NETWORKING

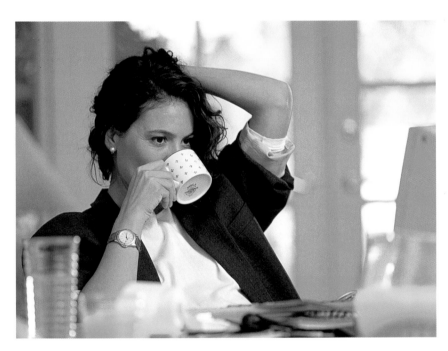

Work that keeps you young. . .

- Work that brings you into contact with new people.
- Work that engages your mind.
- Physically active work.
- Work involving some travel.
- Work you find meaningful.
- Work that requires you to look attractively professional, in which you are expected to be a role model.
- Work you enjoy.

Work that makes you feel old . . .

- Working alone all the time.
- Poorly paid work.
- Work that involves very long hours, with few breaks.
- Constantly shifting work hours.
- Repetitive work which doesn't involve the intellect.
- Work over which you have little control.
- Work where everyone else is a lot older than you.
- Work in a depressing, gloomy building.
- Work that you hate or find boring.

If You've Been Out of the Marketplace for Years

If you haven't worked in a long time and are thinking about rejoining the work force, the first two things you need to focus on are what you would like to do and what action is required to secure such a job. You should also follow the complete 10-week program, because in today's job marketplace your appearance, your health, your confidence levels, and everything else the program has been designed to improve, are all-important in securing that new position you want. If you're competing for a job against 25-year-olds you have many advantages over them– don't spoil your chances by neglecting features such as style, which you have complete control over. This program is intended to make you feel and look wonderful. Use it to help you land a new job and a new career.

Deciding What You'd Like to Do

You may already have a definite idea about what you want to do. That's fine—with one reservation. If it is what you used to do, maybe 10 or 20 years ago, ask yourself. Do I still want to do that? Or am I just going for the safe comfortable option and are there other things I could consider? You aren't the same person you were then; the job probably isn't the same either. So don't rush too quickly into the same type of work – even to the same company – without thinking it through.

If you don't have a definite idea you should think big and then gradually narrow the field down to a few ideas for investigating more thoroughly. Follow this five-point plan:

CASE HISTORY

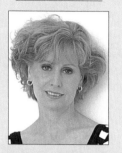

Hilary, 43, got married and had her first baby by the time she was 18.

Three years ago, with Amanda growing up, Hilary realized she had many years ahead of her and wanted to find a career.

"I knew I didn't have the skills necessary to work in an office–I wasn't computer-literate, for example. And anyway, the idea of office life didn't appeal to me."

Instead, Hilary decided that what she really wanted was a career in child care. "I decided to apply for a course to become a day-care nurse. The thought of going to school at my age–then 40–was quite frightening, but I realized that if I didn't train, I wouldn't get the kind of job I wanted. On my first day at college, I passed my lecture hall and felt so daunted I almost didn't go in. But I did–thank goodness–and within a few weeks I felt good about myself. I was proving I still had a brain. Now I have a job I love and the future looks good. When you've spent so long bringing up children it's difficult to readjust when that job is more or less finished. But you can't sit and do nothing. You've got to make a new life for yourself."

Gathering ideas for a new career

1 Decide into which broad area your ideal work fits. For instance, you may want to work in finance. You may want to work in the leisure industry. You may want to work in one of the traditional professions – medicine, law, and so on. You may like the idea of retail sales and marketing. You may want an outdoor job, or one working with children or animals. You may want to break into media, or work in social services. You may want to work from home, and/or start your own business (in which case, see Your Own Business, below). If you're not sure of your area, the library, bookshops, Internet, or local Department of Labor office, will help you. Alternatively, you could enroll in a vocational guidance course. Just because you haven't done something before, doesn't mean you can't start now although the more ambitious you are the more likely it is you will need college or university training/retraining.

2 List your existing talents and interests, and any previous career experience, see how many of them you can employ in your chosen area, or which would help on a job application. If the answer is "nothing" you may have picked the wrong field. If you're still not sure, carry on with steps 3–5.

3 Narrow the field range down to specifics. For example, if you decide you want to work in the leisure industry, do you want to run a hotel, work as a travel agency, or evaluate hotels and vacation destinations for a large travel company? If the latter two ideas appeal to you, it will help if you have extensive experience of travel, staying in hotels, writing reports, and so on.

4 Find out if the type of job you'd like is available in your area. If not, would you move?

5 Research (using the information services listed in point 1) the qualifications you will need for your ideal job, whether you can get them while working your way through a company (age may be an important factor here), or whether you need to study for a specific degree. Write to or call the human resources department of specific companies or trade associations in your chosen field requesting career and training information.

YOUR OWN BUSINESS

Many women dream of running their own business or of working for themselves from home. Here are some ideas to help make that a reality for you:

● Have a clear idea of what you want to do, how you are going to do it, and ensure you have the aptitude, the talent, and the experience for it.

● Research the market.

● Unless you have unlimited funds and enjoy high-level stress, start small. One idea is to start in a very small way while still in other employment–for example, if you want to design and sell knitwear, begin with word of mouth in your spare time. As you get orders, think about advertising, giving up work, and so on.

● If you need financial backing,

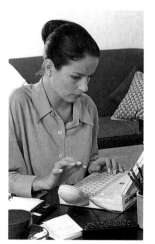

go to the bank with a professional proposal covering your plans for the next two years. Include plenty of information on why there is a need for what you are going to offer.

● Work out of your home if possible – this immediately cuts overhead tremendously.

● If you work from home, it's important to stay in touch with people–not just customers or clients–to stay sane and happy. Make lunch dates with former colleagues; join trade or general organizations for the self-employed or women in business.

Taking Action
Do what you have to do to get that job.

• If you need to retrain or get a degree to qualify, decide whether it is practical for you to do that. Can you afford the time? Can you afford the expense? Investigate this as far as necessary, visiting the educational institution and talking to the financial aid and career advisers.

• If cash is a problem, investigate government-funded programs or private scholarships or tuition reimbursement from the company for which you wish to work.

• Consider working part-time or flextime or doing volunteer work in your chosen profession, especially if you are interested in a job where an immediate full-time paid vacancy is not going to be easy to get. Once you become a familiar face and prove your value you will find your goal easier to achieve.

• If you are qualified for the job you want, but you don't have a specific company in mind, scan the job ads in the newspapers and in trade publications. Apply for jobs you think you may qualify for.

• Get your résumé organized. You can buy books on writing a good résumé or you can pay to have one prepared by one of many companies offering this service. A good résumé writer will work with you and review your background to highlight all your skills and achievements—even those you may have overlooked or forgotten.

• When you get an interview, these few tips will help it go well:

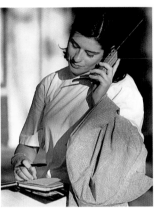

Do your homework! Make sure you know all about the company, and rehearse a two-minute self-presentation highlighting your experience and skills. Make your age a plus, not a minus, by showing maturity, wisdom, experience, self-confidence, poise, and approachability as well as good grooming.

Control nerves by deep-breathing techniques (described on page 110).

Choose an optimum day, if possible, for the interview, such as after a long weekend break when you are fresh and relaxed. Do not schedule the appointment at a bad time, such as before a period if you get PMS, or in the middle of a bad cold.

Wear clothes appropriate for the job—professional, slightly understated clothes that make you feel good are the ideal. Avoid anything uncomfortable or sexy. Neutral colors and navy blue are often good choices.

Have a sense of humor. It's not always easy to strike the right balance, but if you can make the interviewer smile it helps. But your humor should never be at his or her expense or that of the company.

Talk to the interviewer. Remember to make eye contact with the interviewer; listen attentively; ask questions; and most important—smile. It will relax him or her.

If You're Dissatisfied with Your Current Job

Due to the recession, many women I know have stayed in the same job for years, holding to the philosophy that they are lucky to have a job and shouldn't rock the boat by trying for promotion, moving, or trying something totally different. This is a pity. If you use your common sense—and much of the advice above for new job hunters—you can get out of your career rut with minimal risk.

If you are looking for promotion, or perhaps a lateral move within your company, be positive, be confident, be determined, and also keep your ears and eyes open for opportunities to make your wishes known (if appropriate) or to be considered along with other applicants. Seek out opportunities to meet and mingle with company colleagues—business parties, company outings, and so on. Offer to help on special projects. And don't be falsely modest about your achievements. (Don't feel guilty about this, everyone else does it, so you must as well if you are to stand a chance!)

If you are often passed over for promotion in favor of new or younger employees, ask why. Then, if appropriate, work toward improving yourself so next time you won't be overlooked, or discreetly explore the job market. It's best to do this without acrimony because you may need a reference.

If you decide to apply for a completely different type of job, either within your own field or in another, go back to the beginning of this workshop and review the advice for women reentering the job market.

L earning isn't just for the young – all research shows that our brains stay more alert if they are worked and stretched throughout life. If you haven't really learned anything since you were at school or college, now is the time to start educating yourself again.

WORKSHOP 19 EDUCATION

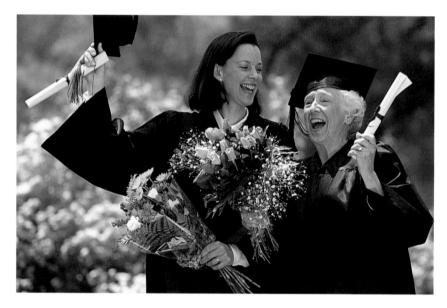

After the frenetic 20s, when you're busy forging a career (and, no doubt, have had enough of books and writing papers for the time being anyway), and the nonstop 30s when you're coping with children as well as work, your middle years can be the perfect time to rediscover your intelligence and set it to work on new subjects.

It has been said that our learning capacity slows down as we get older – for instance, you can learn the basics of a new language in hours at age 12 but at age 50 it may take weeks. While we may not learn as *quickly* as when we were young, our capacity for learning does not diminish. Wanting to learn, being really interested in the subject is the most important criterion for success. Age also has the advantage of experience, and with the self-discipline so often lacking when we are children or young adults.

In this workshop I offer some ideas on what you might like to learn and how you might go about it.

What do you want to know?

• You might like to go back to a subject you liked at school or college and explore it further. Spend a few minutes thinking about what you enjoyed or felt you had an aptitude for. A few ideas include: comparative religion, a science, a language, literature, social history, politics, nutrition. Overview courses are a great way to reintroduce yourself to a subject area.

• You might like to investigate one of the subjects you didn't study before. For instance, when I was at school I remember having to make the choice between history and art. I didn't want to choose between the two but was forced to choose history. In recent years I've tried to make up for that lost subject - not by painting but by studying the lives of some of my favorite artists. Other subjects just weren't around 20 or 30 years ago. What about learning Chinese or doing computer studies, or late 20th century literature?

• Most of us have things we'd like to know more about if we could ever find the time. Now is the time to go through that mental list and pick something that's been a growing interest for the past few years. Maybe interior design or genealogy; maybe botany or theater. (For more practical ideas and more general things, read the next workshop about exploring your own potential.)

A course with a qualification at the end is a goal and a motivation to keep going; however that doesn't suit everyone, and you must decide what you want. Whatever time you have to spare, there are often courses to fit unless you choose something very obscure. Whatever you choose, pick a subject, and a method of learning it, that will give you the end result you want. So it's time to ask yourself a few questions:

- Do I want to learn by myself in my own time and at my own pace?
- Do I want a structured course with a recognized examination and certificate at the end of it?
- Do I just want to do this for fun/satisfaction and don't want a certificate?
- Can I set aside an hour or two/an evening/a day/or more a week to pursue my subject?

For more on practical skills and hobbies, see Workshop 20.

For more on retraining and job skills, see Workshop 18.

If you're going to study you need to bear a few points in mind from the start:

- You need a quiet place to study. Set aside the required amount of quiet time with no outside hassles.
- You need to organize at least a minimal structure for how you study otherwise progress will be erratic.
- Don't study for too long at a time. Your brain will only absorb material well for an hour or two, especially if you are unused to studying or if the subject is difficult. After that length of time, take a meal break or a walk or at the least, work on a different aspect of your subject. As you progress you may find you can study for longer – that's your brain stretching as it is worked, which is where we started!
- Unless you are studying for a qualification in order to get into a new career, you may ask yourself, "What is the point of doing this?" The answer is simple. You are doing this for your own satisfaction, to increase your self esteem by proving you can do it, for pleasure, and because life is for learning. Don't keep the blinkers on.

Going About It

If you're not sure what you want to study, it's always sensible to start by going to your library for information on local courses, classes, and adult education. When you investigate, you might find something that seems interesting that you hadn't thought of before.

- The library will also offer information about organizations, clubs, and societies that might help you further, especially if your chosen subject isn't covered by local courses.
- If you want to study by yourself in your own way and time without a structure, again the library is a good starting point, or your bookshop can provide information about the reading material it has on any specific subject. CD ROM is useful for visuals. The Internet is also useful if you know how to use it.
- If you'd like the structure of an organized class without the pressure of grades, look into the many adult and continuing education classes given through local high schools and colleges.
- If you opt for regular attendance at a class, promise yourself at the beginning that you will attend every lecture. A good way to do this is to pay in advance for a whole session, course, or year.
- Private lessons are another option – good for languages and if you are better on a one-to-one basis or can't travel.

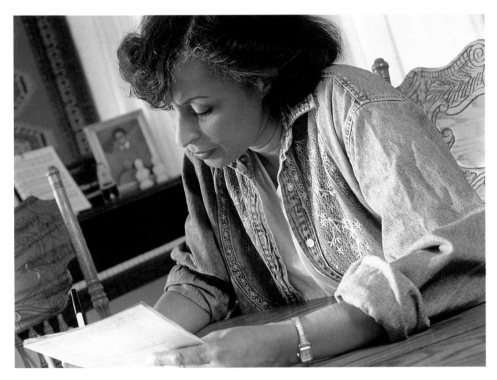

*I*n this workshop, you are to be an explorer. No, that doesn't mean spending your lifesavings on travel or an around-the-world solo tour by elephant. For certain, travel can be a wonderful adventure if you keep your eyes and mind open. Yet many people do travel and discover nothing. However, you can also explore without going too far from home, and that is what this workshop is about–exploring your own potential and life's possibilities. If you lose the ability to question, to search, to keep an open mind, then you're old, whether you're 30 or 100. First try the quiz below.

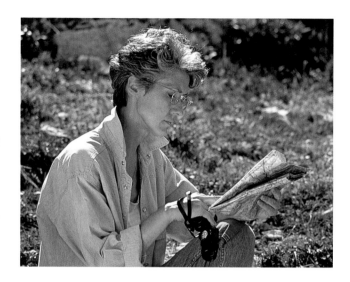

WORKSHOP 20   EXPLORATION

How Open-Minded Are You?

	often	sometimes	never
1 Could you be persuaded to go to a concert or a play that you think you may hate?	❑	❑	❑
2 Do you enjoy being in the company of people more learned, experienced, traveled, or talented than you?	❑	❑	❑
3 On a train, plane, or in a line, do you engage in conversation with a stranger?	❑	❑	❑
4 Do you take time to browse in a library or bookstore?	❑	❑	❑
5 Do you find yourself questioning the way things are traditionally done or the way you have always done things?	❑	❑	❑
6 Do you daydream when you should be working?	❑	❑	❑
7 Do you make decisions based on instinct, not logic?	❑	❑	❑

Check the box for each question, then check your score on the right.

Quiz Results

Now look at your answers. Score 4 for every "often," 2 for every "sometimes," and 0 for every "never." Add your score:

20-28:
You are open-minded, with a great sense of the possibilities of life. You probably don't need this workshop, but I can guarantee you'll read it anyway!

10-19:
You sometimes find yourself wishing you could be more daring. You allow your disciplined side to rule you a little too often and are sometimes afraid to take chances that would have been right. Use this workshop to help you open up.

Under 10:
You tend to have tunnel vision and are a bit too set in your ways. You don't like to move from your chosen path, which means you're missing out on so much that could enrich your life. You may be a little frightened of life, even if you don't admit it. Yes, it is important to be focused and disciplined, but you need balance–use Workshop 15 to help you relax enough to be able to enjoy life and use this workshop to help you see what you might be missing.

10 IDEAS FOR EXPLORERS

Read the ideas that follow thoroughly and apply each one to your life. After you've read them all, make a list of the best ideas for you–and see how many you can fit into your life in the weeks ahead.

1 Keep an open mind.

If you ever find yourself saying things like, "*That* wouldn't be any good!" or "I *never* do that," stop and think. Why wouldn't it be any good? Why don't I try that? You may be right, but don't be too quick to turn down ideas and innovations. Sometimes it is good and invigorating for your well-being to try something new. Also, it is good to occasionally evaluate your views – on politics, religion, or something simple like what food you enjoy. By reviewing yourself and your actions and those of other people close to you (and doing it throughout your life), you keep yourself fresh and up to date. It is so easy just to carry on as you always have because it requires less effort. Once you stop trying to make an effort, however, you start getting old!

2 Keep your eyes open.

People look but often don't see. Start looking around you every day. If you live in the city, notice the architecture where you walk every day. If you live in the country, stop to examine closely the wildflowers. If you used to pay attention to such details, how long since you last did? Would you know what kinds of tree grow on your street? Look at people. You never need to be bored on public transportation if there are other people around. You can play the "people" game: Look at what someone is wearing. Who are they? What do they do? Where are they going?

3 Explore your own capabilities.

In the last workshop we considered how you could return to education–but how about the other areas of your life? When we are young we tend to push ourselves to see what our limits are; as we get older we give up. However, there is no reason to do so. Tell yourself you can do anything you want to do, then decide what that

is. Isn't it time you tried a new hobby or two? Anything from learning to scuba dive or play tennis. . . Write a list now of all the

things you'd like to do. If you're fitter with the help of our exercise and stamina workshops, you can try something new for your body–a new sport or activity, such as dancing, for example.

Or, think of a money-making interest–you could learn to cut hair, propagate plants, or paint. Don't ever sit at home feeling bored–find out what you can do. And don't put up with a dull job–you can cope with a more interesting challenge, so read Workshop 18 and start looking for something better.

4 Explore other people.

Other people's ideas, experiences, and knowledge are gifts you should use as often as possible. If you've stopped listening to people, stopped reading books, stopped asking questions, and become insular–think again. You should read as much as you can, listen as much as you can (but not to bores), and take any opportunity to absorb information that helps you improve your life. By using other people's knowledge and experience, you grow and improve.

5 Explore yourself.

Another way to grow and improve is to delve into your own mind.

Work out what "makes you tick" and you can set about working on your faults, maximizing your good points, improving how

you deal with others, and deciding what you want from your life. It isn't selfish to think about yourself. If you find this hard, there are plenty of self-help books and many self-discovery courses available world-wide.

6 Stop being a spectator.

Get into the habit of joining in, rather than watching. We each watch an average of three hours of television a day. What are your favorite types of program? If you love plays, instead of watching them, why not join a drama club? If you love sports programs, particularly golf and tennis, why not join a golf or tennis club? Do you take your children or grandchildren swimming, but sit there and watch? Join in.

7 Make things happen.

Somebody will–why not you? Far too many of us sit around waiting for other people to organize things, to contact us, to make the first move, for our luck to change. You can make things happen and you can make your own luck. Telephone people. Get involved in local events (the local newspaper may not be literature but it is full of news and ideas about your own area). If you feel bad about local

pollution, fast traffic, or whatever, don't gripe about it–set up an action group.

Believe in things you want and be persistent. You may not get it all, but you'll have more than if you sit and wait and do nothing.

8 Do something different.

Get yourself out of a rut by making a conscious effort to change long-standing patterns of behavior. If your partner always mows the grass, do it yourself. If you always wear black, wear pink. If you always get up at 8 a.m., get up at 4 a.m. on a June day and enjoy the dawn. If you always plan ahead, today go to a bus or train station and decide where you will go on the spur of the moment. And so on. Think of some ideas for yourself. You'll get a real buzz from a small change.

9 Daydream.

Every now and then let your mind wander. You might get some good ideas. The best times to daydream are before you go to sleep, when you wake up (if you don't have to get up immediately), and on a train or plane.

10 Be a silent stranger.

How long has it been since you took yourself off, on your own, to somewhere you've never been before–to somewhere totally new even for an hour? It is a real tonic and a wonderful chance for keeping your mind and eyes open. Find a park and sit and observe. Find a cafe and while away a lunchtime watching people. If you live in a city it's great to go to a different neighborhood and absorb the different atmosphere. How long since you saw the sea? Go there and be a stranger. Get a map and decide where to go. If it helps, pretend you're researching a novel or a play. You may get the inspiration really to do it!

*W*ork and routine often dominate huge chunks of our lives so in time we often forget how very important–and enjoyable–it is to have a good social life. By that I don't mean parties every night, but a circle of friends we trust and with whom we can share. Having friends, and being a good friend, isn't selfish or frivolous. Being a socially integrated person can help keep you young and in touch. Friendship is uplifting, reassuring, revitalizing, and stimulating–all things you need to feel good about yourself. Being a good friend also helps you feel good about yourself; it raises your sense of self-esteem.

WORKSHOP 21

SOCIABILITY

Friendship Quiz

Let's take stock of your social life and see if you can make improvements. First, do this Friendship Quiz. Check the answer that seems to you to be the most truthful.

1 *How many friends do you have with whom you feel completely at ease and to whom you can tell anything?*
- ❏ *a.* None
- ❏ *b.* One or two
- ❏ *c.* Several

2 *How many friends do you have who aren't connected with your work?*
- ❏ *a.* None
- ❏ *b.* One or two
- ❏ *c.* Several

3 *If you had a party, how many people can you think of that you'd really like to see there (and who would be likely to accept)?*
- ❏ *a.* Not enough for a party
- ❏ *b.* Enough for a small party
- ❏ *c.* Enough for a big party

4 *If you were extremely depressed what would you most likely do?*
- ❏ *a.* Sit it out on your own
- ❏ *b.* Telephone a help hotline
- ❏ *c.* Telephone a good friend

5 *How often do you spend a day or evening in the company of friends?*
- ❏ *a.* Less than once a month
- ❏ *b.* Every two or three weeks
- ❏ *c.* At least once a week

6 *Do friends usually telephone you?*
- ❏ *a.* Rarely–you always call them
- ❏ *b.* Always–you don't bother to telephone them
- ❏ *c.* As much as you call them

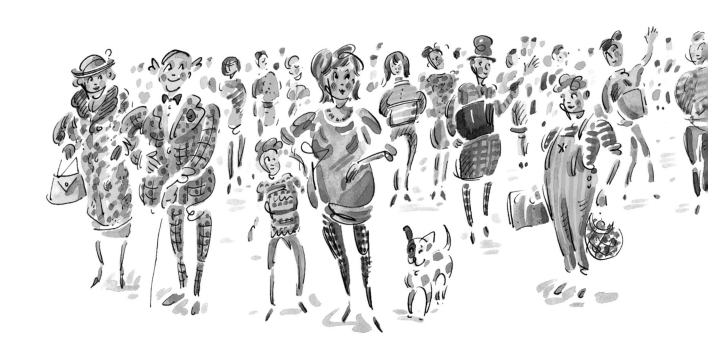

Quiz results

Score 1 for every A, 2 for every B, and 3 for every C you checked.

Add up your score and read your result below.

Over 35:

You're an excellent socializer and no doubt very popular, too. You know how to make friends and how to keep them. And you realize how very important they are in your life. You are just as good at making deep friendships as you are at making time for people passing through. You don't really need to do the rest of Workshop 21 (except for page 129) but you probably will anyway–just for fun!

21-35:

You are unsure of your success socially. Sometimes you think you're doing well and feel secure, with enough people you can rely on, and sometimes you're a terrific friend yourself. You might, however, feel a bit lonely and isolated. Maybe you lead a very busy life and find it hard to fit in the demands friends may make on you. It is worthwhile making that effort, though, so complete the workshop and see what areas of your social life you most need to work on.

20 or under:

You want a good social life and close friends and you recognize the importance of both, otherwise you wouldn't have gotten this far with the workshop. For some reason, however, it isn't working for you. You're likely to lead a solitary life (even if on the surface it doesn't appear that way) and may experience deep bouts of loneliness and even depression. The future could be bleak if you don't let more people into your life and your heart. Carry on with the rest of this workshop and follow up on the ideas.

7 *Are your friends mostly:*

❑ *a.* Friends from ages ago; you have no or few new friends?

❑ *b.* All new friends, you have no or few friends from years ago?

❑ *c.* A mix of old and new friends?

8 *If you move/change jobs, do you keep in touch with the people you've left behind?*

❑ *a.* Rarely

❑ *b.* Occasionally

❑ *c.* A lot

9 *When you feel like going out, can you find someone to go with you (apart from husband, partner, or family)?*

❑ *a.* With difficulty

❑ *b.* Sometimes

❑ *c.* Easily

10 *Do you ever go for days without talking to a friend?*

❑ *a.* Frequently

❑ *b.* Occasionally

❑ *c.* Never

11 *Do you find people boring?*

❑ *a.* Yes, many people

❑ *b.* A few people

❑ *c.* Very few people

12 *Do you remember your friends' birthdays?*

❑ *a.* Rarely

❑ *b.* Sometimes

❑ *c.* Always

13 *Do you have any friends with whom you'd be comfortable seeing you cry?*

❑ *a.* No

❑ *b.* Maybe one

❑ *c.* More than one

14 *At Christmas, how many cards do you get, excluding relatives and business cards?*

❑ *a.* Hardly any

❑ *b.* Quite a few

❑ *c.* Dozens

10 WAYS TO FIND NEW FRIENDS

❶ Don't be too reserved and don't always expect other people to initiate a friendship. If you like the look or sound of someone, talk to him/her, find out what he/she likes and when the time is right make a casual invitation based on what you know. For example, if a woman likes gardening, suggest she might like to come along with you to a garden open to the public.

❷ Share your interests by joining a club. Singing, acting, gardening, painting, whatever you enjoy there is a club to join. Haven't got any interests? Of course you do (and Workshops 20 and 24 will help you).

❸ Alternatively, start a club of your own–a hobby club, a dining club, a theater club, whatever.

❹ Get active in your community or church.

❺ Ask for help. People like being helpful.

❻ Offer help. If you're good at something other people want to learn, offer your help. Let people know you're glad to help.

❼ Enroll in a continuing education course or go back to college and get that degree.

❽ If your work is isolating, do volunteer work at your local school or hospital or other organization.

❾ The Internet is a great place to "meet and chat" with people who have similar interests.

❿ Slow down. If you're always in a hurry without time to stop and chat you could lose many opportunities for making friends.

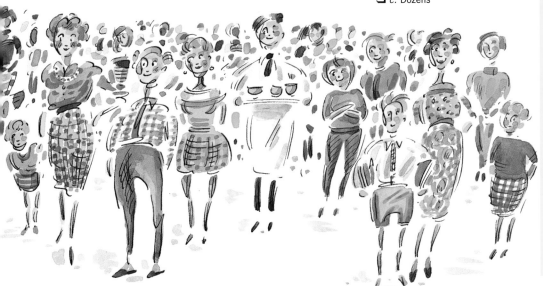

HOW TO KEEP FRIENDS HAPPY

- Telephone regularly.
- Don't feel snubbed if sometimes friends are busy with other things.
- Don't always moan–be cheerful at least some of the time.
- Don't tell any lies other than the occasional white lie, and if you do, ask yourself how you could have avoided the white lie.
- Don't be afraid to show your vulnerable side, your failings, and your failures.
- Listen to your friends.
- Only offer advice if you're asked–and then be very careful, especially about saying anything negative about your friend's partner, family, other friends and aquaintances, and so on.
- Remember birthdays.
- Pay your way, and never borrow anything without returning it or replacing it.
- Be positive. In most situations you can say something either negative or positive; the positive is nearly always the right thing to say.
- Don't burden friends too heavily. You cannot reasonably expect them to be there for you every minute of every day at a second's notice.
- Don't expect one friend to want to share all your interests. That's why a circle of friends is a good idea.
- Remember to give as well as take.

Shyness or reserve or the inability to make initial "small talk" can be a barrier to making friends. But this needn't be so. Most good friendships are built through a common interest, whether it is work, having children at the same school, living in the same apartment building or sharing a hobby.

Sometimes our lack of a social circle is simply because the life we lead doesn't offer opportunities to meet people. For example, someone who has recently moved from a city to the country and works from home will have to make an effort to go places and do things to make friendships happen.

The box on page 123 gives you 10 good ways to meet or encourage people who may become friends. Not all the ideas will be possible for you, but some *will* work.

Making new friends in the middle years is a wonderful challenge, filled with the possibilities of adventure. It's never too late to start.

How to Keep Friendship Alive

By the time we reach our 30s and older, most of us have had many friends in our lives. Most of us, too, have lost as many friends. Obviously, it's almost impossible to stay friends with every person you've known, but to keep a proportion of

Making Friends

your friends throughout life is enriching and even more important than having the knack to get a new friendship off the ground.

Do you like people?
I know someone who goes through "friends" at an alarming rate–the fallout is tremendous. She will drop someone for any small reason–for example, being late to meet her; not agreeing with her; forgetting to pass on a piece of gossip; or saying something critical.

To be a good friend you need to give as much as you take, and you have to like your friends and be interested in their lives. Even more important, you need to accept them with their failings.

No one is perfect, so don't discard people before you've honestly asked yourself, "Am I expecting too much?" If you wait for the perfect friend, you'll die waiting.

Do people like you?
What is it that makes one person say of another person, "I don't like her!" or, "I could never be friends with her!"?

Generally, saying we don't like someone translates to, "That person makes me feel negative about myself in some way." We don't like people who make us feel inferior, stupid, dull, invisible, jealous, and so on.

If you think you are more likely to be popular if you always have the latest car, live in the best house, wear nothing but designer clothes, never have a hair out of place, and always want the last word, you couldn't be more wrong. You are only likely to intimidate people. Make people feel good about themselves and you will surely be the most

popular person around.

Review the box on How to Keep Friends Happy (left). Ask yourself if you do those things at least some of the time. If not, now is the time to begin being a better friend.

Finding a Soul Mate

Your partner may be a soul mate but few things beat having someone who isn't a lover to talk to about everything. If you are lucky enough to have such a person in your life, recognize his or her importance to you and cherish that friendship. You can't conjure up such friends to order. If you follow all the tips in this workshop, however, you will put yourself in line for finding one. Usually when we meet a soul mate, we know almost instantly. You start talking and never stop, and friendship seems natural from that moment. Nothing is forced, there is no need to try. That kind of closeness is very special. It doesn't mean you will never argue or annoy each other, but it is true, deep friendship.

Sometimes your soul mate is harder to detect–it may even be the person about whom you said, "I could never be friends with her!" Underneath that arrogant, perfect, untouchable, or superior facade may be the loneliest, but nicest, person around. Never give up on people until you've tried. Sometimes the best friends come well disguised.

Your Family Matters

Do you have a family. . . parents, brothers, sisters, children, grandchildren, cousins, uncles, aunts. . . ? If you do, do you enjoy them and appreciate them enough? Sadly, many of us don't. For some of us, lack of close family contact is a result of the way many of us have lived our lives so far:

• Leaving our family home or area to get the education and then the job we wanted removed us from family.

• Many of us have divorced and thus fragmented the family further.

• Maybe we had our children cared for by other people most of the time and don't feel as involved with them now as we would like.

• Or perhaps we were so busy building our careers and our nest eggs that keeping close contact with family didn't seem so important.

• We might have had our children later than our mothers and grandmothers; our own children are having their children late, too—meaning we all have to wait later for grandchildren, nephews, nieces, and so on.

The result of any of these? We've got out of the habit of closeness with family, and, whether we choose to admit it or not, that can lead to loneliness, loss of support, feelings of guilt, and most important, loss of pleasure and a sense of belonging. Women now in their late 30s, 40s, and early 50s are the first generation of women to realize that demanding careers and modern society come with a price. Of course, this isn't true for all of us, but it is true of a surprisingly high number.

And for those of us who didn't go that route and do have a family nearby, many

of us quite simply take that family for granted. We may even complain about them.

Whether you have distant family, fragmented family, or family in proximity you don't appreciate, think of the millions of people who

aren't lucky enough to have any sort of family. You can make friends, but you can't make family. So you should realize how fortunate you are to have blood relations, and start making friends of them.

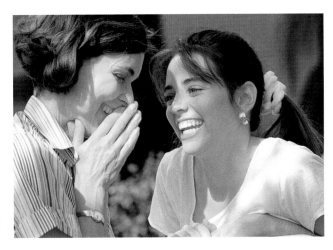

Family checklist

If your family is far away

• Telephone regularly.

• Write regularly.

• Send and ask for photos, videos, and tapes to keep in touch better.

• Visit whenever you can. Don't automatically put family last on your list; is work really more important?

• Invite them to visit whenever you can. If you're busy, make sure they help; treat them like family, rather than guests.

If your family is near

• Look at their good points rather than their failings.

• Count your blessings.

• Have regular arranged times when you will visit them and they will visit you.

• Be on the lookout for relatives who need help. Many are too proud to ask. If you can't help them, who can?

• And don't be too proud yourself to ask for help or admit life isn't going well. Your family can provide the best shoulders to cry on, even better than friends.

• Try your best to be friends with your ex-husband, and/or your partner's family.

• Make as much time as you can for your children and grandchildren, especially when they are young. It's valuable time. Women tend to regret missing those early years most.

Whether your family is close or distant

• Make allowances. Use the same principles in the "How to Keep Friends Happy" box on your relatives as well.

• If you have an argument, make up. I have a friend who hasn't seen her only sister for 10 years after an argument about a borrowed outfit. Most family arguments are over petty things that aren't worth falling out over.

• Show appreciation. If you can't say it, write it.

• Tell yourself you're lucky. If you want confirmation that you are, look around–you'll soon have your confirmation.

*I*f you have been with the same partner for a decade or more you may find that some of the early passion, fun, and spontaneity have gone from your relationship. It's time to see what can be done.

WORKSHOP 22 RELATIONSHIPS 1 – LONG-TERM LOVE

However slim, fit, and energetic you feel toward the end of your 10-week program, it is difficult to feel as fresh and alluring as a 20-year-old on her first date if you are in a long-term relationship that is hovering somewhere between the predictable and the downright stale. There is also perhaps nothing as aging, mentally, as the realization that your partner thinks you are about as sexy as a pair of old slippers (or vice versa).

But this workshop isn't just about sex, it's about enjoying your partner–and life with your partner–again. That said, if you're like most women you will want an enjoyable sex life. Research shows good sex keeps you young, so let's start from that point.

"Our Sex Life Isn't Great"

I hate all those articles in women's magazines about how to revive your sex life with your partner by wearing frilly underwear and exotic perfume, or cooking his favorite supper by candlelight while wearing little else. It is hardly subtle, and it hardly ever works. Your partner would probably think you have gone slightly crazy and feel embarrassed, and you (I fear) would feel ridiculous. You'd be better off watching a sexy movie together.

The fact is, however, that if you've been involved with someone for a long time it is almost impossible to recreate the exhilaration you felt in the early months of the relationship. That feeling lasts only a few years or so if you're lucky. By the time you hit your tenth wedding anniversary or later, the only way to get that feeling back is to fall in love with someone else. However, that is not to say you can't enjoy good sex with your mate. Here's how:

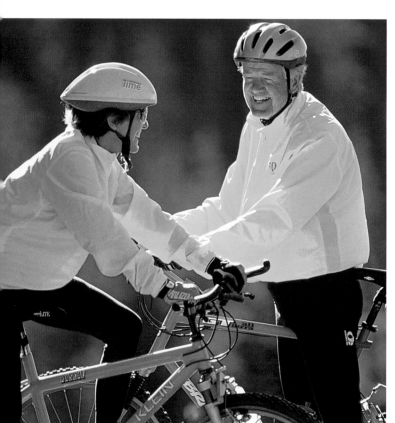

- Make sure you like each other. If one or both of you is filled with underlying resentment or misery, you're not really going to look forward to sex. Talk about problems and, if you can't, consider counseling.

- Be nice to him, and if he is nice to you, make sure he knows you appreciate it.

- Keep fit and active and organize your days, both of you (see Workshop 12), so you aren't exhausted every night when you climb into bed, or set the alarm a bit earlier than usual in the mornings, or find another time of day when you can make love.

- Take regular time apart from each other. Many couples live in constant contact with each other, then wonder why they feel bored.

- Keep yourselves evolving– Workshop 21 is full of ideas– rather than stagnating. You may find him much sexier if you see him in a new light. Flirting helps here, too. If he sees you in conversation with another man he too will see you afresh.

- A sexy video before bed really can help get you both in the mood.

- Do enjoyable things together at least some of the time.

CASE HISTORY

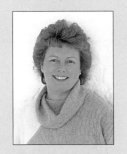

Pamela has been married to her husband Nick for 30 years, and she puts the success of her marriage down to several factors:

"I didn't marry until I was 27, and by that time I had traveled a lot, done and seen plenty, and so was quite ready for the commitment of marriage. Secondly, Nick and I were great friends before we began dating, and I think that is very important – he is still my best friend!

"I think divorce is too easy now, so often I see people split up almost at the first sign of problems; you have to realize that you are two different people and won't always agree; work things out rather than give up easily. With the next partner there are going to be problems too. Nick and I have had our upsets, but you learn to accept your differences.

"And to keep boredom at bay and your marriage alive it is important that you both have your own interests and not spend every moment together. You've also got to keep communicating and not neglect your husband for the children. When they have gone he's the one your going to be stuck with after all!"

Evolving in Your Relationship

I know several women who have divorced attractive, kind, hard-working, generous, healthy husbands for no better reason than that 20 or so years after the wedding, the excitement and passion had disappeared. They mostly went off with younger men and some, after two or three years in a new marriage, are again feeling dissatisfied because the exhilaration of being "in love" is already fading. . . even faster than it did the first time.

You have to choose among making a deep and ever-evolving relationship, having serial marriages or partners, or being on your own. For those who manage it, the former is undoubtedly the most rewarding and enriching, and it always amazes me how so many couples split up so lightly after sharing such a lot.

With a successful relationship you simply and gradually replace the things that held you together in your first years—lust, newness, excitement, insularity, and so on, with new things—parenting, friendship, caring, shared interests, a sense of your own history, and so on. You can't have it both ways—but the things that come with time are even better.

Does any of this apply to you? If you're feeling slightly bored and discontent, slightly stale with your relationship, and half looking for something better, try to see the good things about it.

• Make a list of all the good points about your relationship together.

• Make a list of all the good points about your partner's personality.

• Make a list of all the good aspects of your life in general. Try also to think through whether your boredom has as much to do with too little going on in the rest of your life as it does with your partner.

• Do you have platonic friends? (See Workshop 19.)

• Is your job satisfying–or, if you don't have one, should you get one? (See Workshop 18.)

• Is your personal life fulfilling? (See Workshop 21.)

When someone is always around it is easy to assume he or she will always be around, and stop trying to work on growing the relationship. However, a close, long-lasting relationship is a prize to be cherished. It's so easy to let it go due to carelessness . . . and so hard, to get another. So be as certain as you can be before you tell him it's over.

"Should I Dump Him?"

We all have the odd day when we could murder our partners – they feel the same. There's no such thing as a perfect relationship all the time. It's all compromise. However, if you're living in a relationship that is making you chronically unhappy, you don't have to stay. No amount of diet and exercise can take 10 years off your looks if you're miserable. Unhappiness is the most aging emotion, and there is a time to admit defeat and let go. If you stayed for the kids, and now they're grown; if he's had one affair too many; if he's a bully, or violent . . . don't feel sorry for him and stay. Take charge of your life.

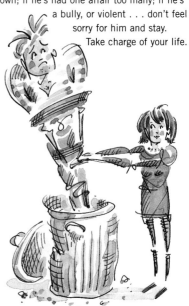

This checklist may help you decide:

1 Is it him who is making you unhappy? Is your own behavior at fault, too? If so, are either of you prepared to try to alter your behavior? Can you compromise more? Can you settle for less? Do you want to?
2 Does he know how you feel? Have you tried to tell him? Have you succeeded? Would counseling help?
3 If you still think you should end the relationship, try visualizing your life after the split. If you can visualize your future life and feel positive about it, then you should end it. Maybe a "trial separation" would be possible. If you've lived with someone a long time, an uncertain future can seem almost as bad as a terrible relationship – but you owe it to yourself

So you're divorced, separated, widowed, or never a permanent partner. For whatever reason, you're on your own and you're out of practice. But you don't want to be on your own. Quite right. Living alone may be peaceful and blissfully selfish and tidy, but good sex and good love keep you young–it's a well-documents fact. However, you don't have to live with him to enjoy both of those. You're wise enough and independent enough now to need a man only for the pleasures he can offer you. In this workshop you'll find some ideas for finding and keeping that man.

WORKSHOP **23** # RELATIONSHIPS 2
STARTING AGAIN

Where Do You Look?

It is often said that if you're looking for a partner you won't find him, but when you stop looking you will. This is partially true– desperation is obvious and extremely unappealing, and should be avoided at all costs. However, there isn't any harm in looking in a relaxed kind of way. Hoping to meet someone just by chance is likely to involve you in a long wait.

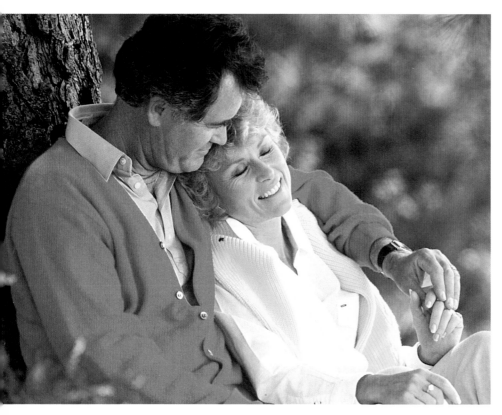

Where to look? First a list of "nos"–meeting places that aren't ideal for the newly single mature woman who's out of practice dating and is vulnerable. Some of these, however, may be fine for a different sort of person; it's a subjective list.

✗ **NO** to singles bars. They are far too depressing, unsafe, and usually make anyone over the age of 25 feel ancient.

✗ **NO** to night clubs. A few are suitable for older women to go to with a couple of friends, but if you don't choose well you're likely to end your evening feeling very miserable.

✗ **NO** to personal ads. Whether you put your own ad in the paper or reply to someone else's, it can be an extremely soul-destroying way to find someone you even like, let alone are attracted to. It can also be dangerous. If you insist on trying, pick a reputable paper or magazine that is read by people like yourself, make initial meetings only in public places, and stay very, very cynical.

✗ **NO** to the workplace. Trying to start a relationship at work can be difficult and is rarely wise, whether it's the boss, your assistant, or the office "go-fer." If you approach him and get rebuffed, or have a relationship that goes wrong, it will cause problems.

✗ **NO** to dating services, where you pay an annual fee and are put in touch with a

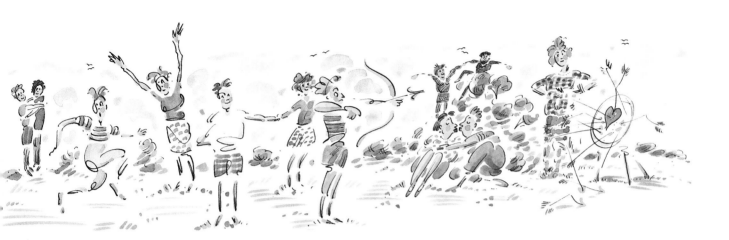

"suitable" partner on a one-to-one basis. This may not be a source of danger, but it is certainly almost as soul-destroying as the personal ads. After six months of being offered "Mr. Rights," who are definitely wrong, your confidence in yourself and in men will likely be zero.

✗ NO to your best friend's partner. It's surprising how often this happens. You'll have better success following the tips below. Nine out of ten women who follow this path lose both their friend and the man, eventually.

That may not appear to leave many places to look, but it does. The major point to bear in mind is that once you're past the age for discos and hanging out with your friends on the street, most couples meet in a group situation or while going about normal life. Occasionally it's love at first sight, but more often you slowly get to love each other. Bearing this in mind let's look at some likely "yes" places to meet.

✔ Yes to private parties, weddings, and so on. You have a chance to look stunning and be among people you know, so you aren't nervous and there is always someone you can talk with. But never have more than two drinks.

✔ Yes to blind dates set up by friends. You should be able to trust your friends to choose, if not someone to whom you're instantly attracted, then at least someone you like well enough to see as a friend.

✔ Yes to any hobby or club that really does interest you. There's no point joining the local gym in the hope of meeting a hunk if you can't even lift a two-pound weight and don't want to–you'll feel and look like an idiot. But if you love walking, tennis, photography, or whatever, join a club. Even if you don't find a date there, you will make friends with people who may know other people. And if you're single, you need friends.

✔ Yes to a singles social group. These are growing fast all over the world as people find it harder and harder to meet other single people through the old-style channels. These clubs hold weekly meetings and regular events, such as theater visits, dinners, barbecues, picnics, and so on, and are ideal for meeting a group of like-minded people.

✔ Yes to special interest vacations–some are geared especially for single and/or older people. Ask your travel agent. If you pick an activity you enjoy–biking or photography, for example–you don't have to spend hours on your own by the pool feeling lonely. Again, you may not meet a lover but if you spend your vacation locked inside your apartment you won't meet one, either. At least on an activity vacation you'll

have fun, which is all part of rehabilitating yourself in the "outside world," especially if you've been cloistered with the same partner for years.

Remember, wherever you go be friendly, and first look for companionship. Show your interest in life and in others. If you like someone, let that be a wonderful start. After all, the sexiest man in the world isn't going to make you happy for long if you don't like him.

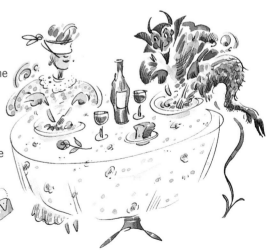

Sex–The New New Etiquette

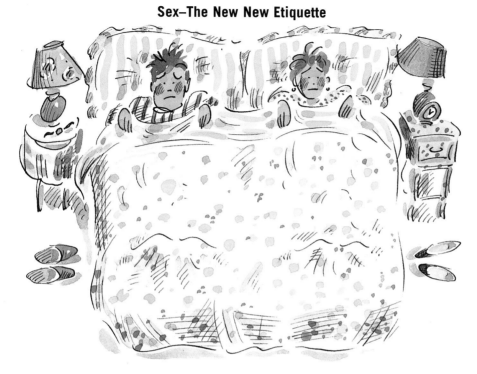

If it has been a while (like 10 or 20 years!) since you had sex with anyone new, there are a few important things you'll need to know.

• It is okay to say no at any stage of love-making, but if you don't want sex, say so as soon as possible. If you don't want sex, make your wishes clear. Even better, before you get into kissing, have a conversation with him about sex and what you want at the moment. If you have already told him that you'd need to know someone very well before sleeping with them, and he gets heavy on the first date, then he's not being fair and you should say so. Or it may be that *you* want sex early in the relationship and he doesn't, which is not as uncommon as you might think. In that case, it's your turn to be patient.

• If you're worried, talk to your physician, a counselor, or a health agency regarding "safe sex" guidelines.

• Intercourse without a condom is a risky activity. Be prepared and expect your partner to use a condom without complaint.

• Don't take offence if he asks if you've been HIV-tested. You might like to ask him, too–but it is better to get this kind of official business out of the way before you get as far as the bedroom.

• You are not only allowed, but expected, to say what you like done to your body and what you would like to do to his. Silence under the covers is no longer the norm. Neither is turning the lights off–so continue working out.

• Don't fake orgasms. If you'd been doing so for years with your previous partner, take this as a great opportunity to change your thinking. What makes a man a great lover is your telling him what you want and how you're feeling. You can't assume that even an experienced man knows exactly how to turn you on. Maybe he's been with the same partner for years who's been faking, too–so you can't blame him for getting it wrong. Don't fake–talk! And if you can't talk, perhaps it's too early to be having sex–a piece of advice every mother gives to her teenage daughter, but is true at any age.

Help! I've Forgotten How to Flirt

When you meet someone you are attracted to you'll probably find it comes easily, or you don't need to even think about flirting, which is even better. Flirting is not always a good thing. It is good if the man you like is obviously shy, if your natural mode is aloof or retiring, and if neither of you are ever going to get together unless someone gives out signals. In other words, mild flirting shows you're interested. It is, however, a bad thing if you overdo it. There's nothing worse to behold than a 45-year-old woman being much too coquettish and coy; he'll run a mile if he's a regular guy.

• On balance, it's best to be mysterious and offer something of a challenge if you have to play games at all. Sexist though it may be, it's true–most men like to think they are doing some chasing. That's not to say you can't be friendly. You should be.

• Smile and laugh and look into his eyes when you're with him; but don't act as if your life –even your evening–depends on him.

• At a party, keep circulating.

• At dinner, talk to the person on your other side.

• Let him call you slightly more than you call him.

• Leave the answering machine on some of the time.

• You want to avoid even a hint of desperation; so if you have even the vaguest feeling that your flirting is bordering on desperate–stop.

Can I Ask Him Out?

Yes, of course you can. However, if you are feeling vulnerable, have never before asked a man, and don't wish to experience what all men have experienced–someone turning you down and making you feel like digging a hole down to the center of the earth–it's wise to follow a few basic precautions:

• Have tickets to something (a football game, the theater) to have in front of him–"Look, I've just been given these. I know you like football/theater–do you want to come along?" Yes, it's corny, but if he really does like the football game/theater he'll most likely accept–unless he can't stand you. If this is the case, you haven't read the signals correctly. If he wants to turn you down, he just has to say, sorry, he's busy that night, and you believe him. If it's true, he'll know you like him and may well ask you to something else at another time.

• It is also good to invite someone out as if to help you out of a spot. "Look, I've been invited to a party but I don't want to go alone, as I only know the host. Will you come with me?"

• Always have a purpose in mind for your date apart from the obvious. It isn't a good idea to just invite him out to dinner at a restaurant or to invite him around to dinner at your place, out of the blue.

• If you're not sure of his interest in you, a daytime date is always the sure bet. It seems less predatory to say, "Come for a picnic with me (and the kids?) in the park if you're not doing anything this weekend!" That way, if he says no, it's no big deal.

In any event, if you follow the guidelines on pages 132 and 133 for where to meet someone, by the time you know you want to date him you'll probably not have to worry about how to arrange a date anyway . . . it will all follow naturally.

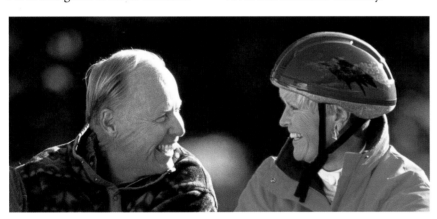

Conquering First Date Nerves

Nervous? Don't worry about it! Just say, "I feel nervous, I haven't had a date with someone new in a long time." If he is the kind of man you are going to like, that will be fine. He's probably nervous, too. If you meet someone first as a friend or through a common interest, first-date nerves won't be a factor because conversation will be easy and things will evolve naturally.

Anyhow, if your new date is someone with whom you can be yourself, your nerves will be short-lived. If he isn't–the relationship may never get off the ground. If he's still making you nervous after a few dates, it might be time for second thoughts.

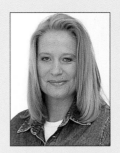

CASE HISTORY

Kay: Two years ago Kay was divorced from her husband to whom she had been married for nearly 20 years, and was in no rush to meet someone new. "It has taken me the two years to adjust to living on my own, and to come to terms with what happened," she says. "I'm still in no rush, which I think is the best way, but now I can start to say, "We shall see!

"I think what you say is right–that if you are totally out of practice at "dating," the very idea can be daunting–and it is much better to try to build up a network of friends, some of whom may happen to be male. Halfway through the 10-week program I began a college course two days a week, which has been wonderful socially as well. I'm going out to parties now and have met quite a few nice men. And now that I am looking better, of course I'm finding a bit more interest. I'm enjoying my freedom–and it will take a special man to change that in the near future."

*H*ow long has it been since you really enjoyed yourself? When was the last time you experienced pure, unadulterated pleasure without a hint of duty or compromise?

24 PURE PLEASURE

I asked several acquaintances those questions and they all had to stop and think hard to remember such an occasion. Three couldn't remember one at all, a fact I find very sad. Nobody could remember the last time they laughed until they cried; nobody could think of a whole evening spent in pure self-indulgence. What pleasures there were, were moments or minutes, rather than hours or days. The longer pleasures cited–visits to the hairdresser by one woman, and a clothes shopping trip by another–came with some guilt attached, along with some unwanted negatives (worrying whether the hairdresser was going to do the style right; busy shops, unhelpful salespeople, and not finding clothes to fit on the shopping trip). So, in fact, they weren't pure pleasure after all.

Women, it seems, are usually programmed to put everyone and everything else in life first. Pleasure comes last, or not at all. Yes, you say you get pleasure from work done well, pleasure from seeing your family enjoy themselves, pleasure from cooking a terrific meal, passing an exam. That's pleasure, but it is, of course, tempered with responsibility or some other restraining emotion.

What we are bad at is hedonistic pleasure–pleasure as a beginning and an end in itself. In other words, FUN! However great your life is, however much it is going according to plan, well organized, and without hassle, if you're not having any fun, what's the point?

You need to be carefree, laugh, giggle, indulge yourself–even in small doses–on a regular basis. And you need to do this without guilt. If you feel guilty, you're not having fun. You have no need to feel guilty. Pure pleasure is not, ironically, just selfish self-indulgence. There are scientifically sound reasons why you should loosen up and enjoy yourself:

● Laughter increases the amount of oxygen in your bloodstream, helping you to feel more energetic and alert.
● Laughter can lower blood pressure and improve both circulation and metabolism.
● Laughter releases endorphins in the body, which are natural pain-killers.
● Laughter boosts the immune system. So laughter may really be "the best medicine."

You don't have to laugh out loud to benefit from times of pure pleasure. When you are enjoying yourself you are:

Mentally more relaxed–stress levels diminish and when you get back to your "responsible" life, you tackle it much better.

Physically more relaxed–facial lines smooth out, digestive problems diminish, and after an enjoyable day or evening you are much more likely to get a good night's sleep. The effect is an upward spiral.

Recharging your batteries–a period of real relaxed enjoyment will always help you to carry out tasks with renewed enthusiasm.

So let's make Workshop 24 a "funshop"; let's kill the guilt and let's examine some ways you can be a hedonist and have pure pleasure without a purpose!

Retrogress...

If you've got out of the habit of enjoying yourself you'll need to psych yourself into it. One of the easiest ways is to think back–maybe even as long ago as your teens; certainly back to your 20s. Think about what you loved to do then, what made you happy, what made you laugh. Now do it again! Have a retro couple of hours. Dig out the old music tapes; look at old photo albums, rent the film or TV series you loved the most. You may not still think it is all terrific, of course – but it's the feeling of what it was like to be carefree and indulgent you are trying to get back. Everyone should relish their past and take time to reminisce now and again. It's soul food.

HEDONISM EXERCISE

Make your own list of pleasures, large or small. If you are out of practice you may have to think for awhile; but the more you do it the easier it becomes. Once the list is made, begin indulging yourself. Enjoy your pleasures–but don't forget the rules:

Include nothing except your own, true, real, deep pleasures.

Don't let other people or outside influences dissuade you. *You are as important as anyone else is.*

Don't feel guilty for your pleasure time. Feel guilty if you *don't* have it!

Progress. . .

Set aside regular pleasure time and fill it with whatever makes you feel good. *Here are some ideas:*

If you have a few days to spare–
● Take the vacation you have always wanted to take but your partner wasn't interested in.

● Spend a few days in bed with TV, or a few novels, and some food that you love and always feel too guilty to eat.

● Spend a few days in bed with your lover.

● Visit a health spa and get as many body massages, facials, and treatments as time and your budget allows.

If you have a few hours to spare–
● Attend the opera/ballet/film/play you've always wanted to see and didn't.

● Watch all the reruns of your favorite TV shows.

● Rent videos of your favorite comedian or book tickets for a live show.

● Read, read, read–for enjoyment, not studying.

● Spend an evening with your favorite friend.

● Drop what you're doing on a perfect day, and take a slow walk in one of your favorite places.

If you have an hour or less to spare–
● Have a bath and a glass of champagne.

● Walk around the garden, taking time to smell the flowers, watch the insects, listen to the birds, soak up the atmosphere.

● Sit in a comfortable chair in a park or garden with your eyes shut.

● Make a phone call to the friend who always makes you laugh.

● Treat yourself to a full body massage.

OUR PARTICIPANTS

JUST LOOK AT THEM NOW!

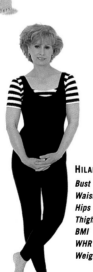

HILARY 10 WEEKS AGO
She stuck to drab, safe colors, and had not changed her hair or makeup for years.

10 WEEKS AGO
Bust 35 inches
Waist 29½ inches
Hips 37½ inches
Thighs 23 inches
BMI 25.5
WHR .79
Weight 145 pounds

HILARY NOW
Bust 35½ inches
Waist 25 inches
Hips 35½ inches
Thighs 21 inches
BMI 23.3
WHR .70
Weight 133 pounds

Hilary, 43, finished the 10-week program weighing 133 pounds– a 12-pound weight loss, and dead on target. At 5ft 4½ inches, her BMI is now 23.3 and her WHR ratio just .70.

"The best thing about the program for me has been the change in my body shape and my fitness level. I can swim 30 lengths instead of one, and could probably do more. My legs have never been so slim in my life, and I even like my knees now. I am wearing short skirts, for the first time. Doing regular exercise has changed so many other things though, too – I have energy, I am less lethargic, but more relaxed and calmer altogether. My PMS symptoms have improved dramatically, too.

"I enjoyed the diet and I virtually never crave sweet things any more. My skin is better and I have learned some makeup tips from Celia I can practice. I love my new hairstyle and so does everyone else–it's so easy to look after.

"The 10-week program was by no means easy all the way through, especially those early weeks of exercise. Now I'm facing the future with much more confidence, and I feel terrific."

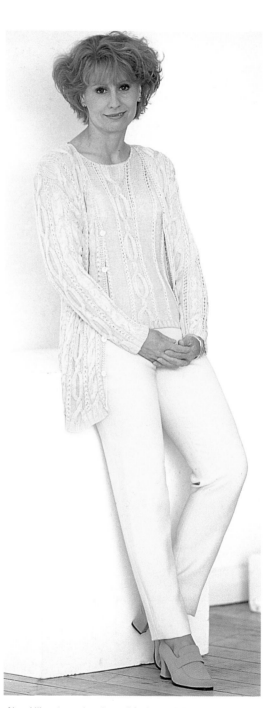

Now Hilary turns heads–and feels much less stressed and more energetic.

Sue's found her true personality–strong and bright –and an image to match it.

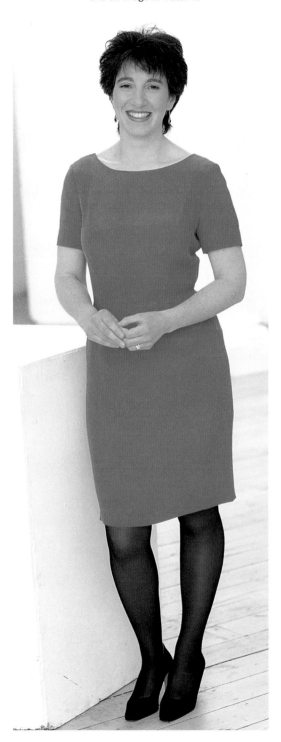

W hen we first met Sue, 39 and 5ft 4 inches, she seemed a shy person for a doctor, almost mouselike. As the weeks progressed, however, we realized there was far more to Sue. Her unshakable determination and strong character began to emerge, and with them, her firm, well-toned, fit new body. Finally, we helped her find her new, bright style to match the rest–and that was it . . . a new, rejuvenated Sue.

"I enjoyed it all," she says, "but particularly having the motivation to do regular exercise. At last I'm as fit as my husband, Steve, now; we've even started going for long cycle rides together. And I don't feel a bit of a fraud when I tell my patients to exercise and to eat healthily any more!

"Actually, I have very much enjoyed changing my eating habits; I feel better psychologically and physically for it. I think it is because of diet as much as the exercise that I feel more energetic throughout the day. I used to suffer from headaches, but even they have diminished. Eating fewer calories was fine–I never felt really hungry or lacking in energy as people often say they do on diets. I ended up losing 14 pounds altogether–slightly lower than the target we set. I won't lose any more, though, as I don't want to be too thin.

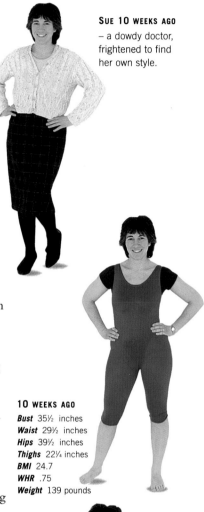

SUE 10 WEEKS AGO
– a dowdy doctor, frightened to find her own style.

10 WEEKS AGO

Bust 35½ inches
Waist 29½ inches
Hips 39½ inches
Thighs 22¼ inches
BMI 24.7
WHR .75
Weight 139 pounds

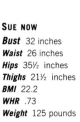

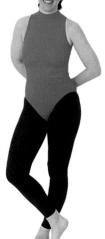

SUE NOW

Bust 32 inches
Waist 26 inches
Hips 35½ inches
Thighs 21½ inches
BMI 22.2
WHR .73
Weight 125 pounds

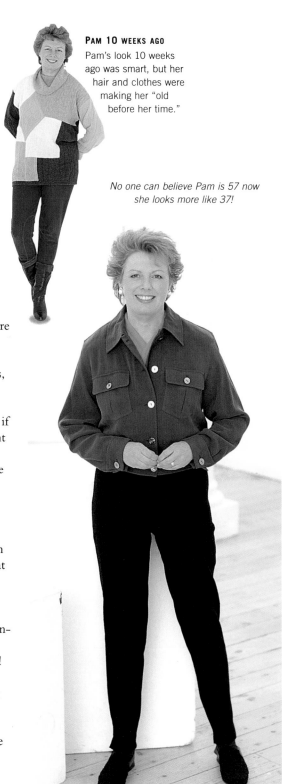

PAM 10 WEEKS AGO
Pam's look 10 weeks ago was smart, but her hair and clothes were making her "old before her time."

No one can believe Pam is 57 now she looks more like 37!

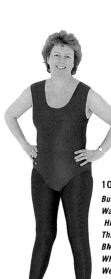

10 WEEKS AGO

Bust 38½ inches
Waist 34½ inches
Hips 40 inches
Thighs 21½ inches
BMI 25.3
WHR .86
Weight 147 pounds

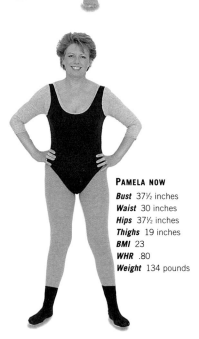

PAMELA NOW

Bust 37½ inches
Waist 30 inches
Hips 37½ inches
Thighs 19 inches
BMI 23
WHR .80
Weight 134 pounds

Pamela has always taken a pride in her appearance–buying top-quality clothes, getting her hair done regularly, enjoying good food, and generally enjoying life. However, 10 weeks ago, overweight and unfit, with her hair in a typical 50s-plus cut and perm, her dress sense ultra-conservative, and her makeup not doing her justice, Pam knew she could do better–she just needed some help.

Now she has lost 13 pounds and taken her BMI and her WHR to within recommended levels–a marvelous achievement. Perhaps more important is the fact that after years of little exercise and a poor level of muscle tone, stamina, and suppleness, Pam, 5ft 5 inches, is now fitter than she's been in her life. This proves it really *is* never too late to start, even if you are taking hormone replacement therapy, as she is.

Pam says, "I am delighted with the results–so many people have commented on how I look. Even my husband likes it–and he hates me to change! My skin and my energy levels are better, and, of course, I can wear so many more clothes now that my waist has shrunk. I could hardly believe how much difference the exercise made to my body. At first I couldn't manage more than a few minutes of exercise without stopping – now I can sail through a whole hour!

"I shall keep up with the exercise and with my healthier eating–doing both means I can still eat out and entertain more or less when I want to, without having to worry that the pounds will pile back on."

A similar sort of look—but what a difference!

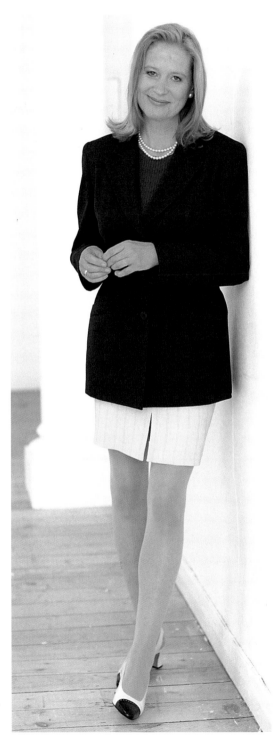

When Kay began the program, to be honest, I wasn't sure that she would come through well. When she tried to exercise, she couldn't follow even basic moves properly and didn't appear to be putting a lot of effort into them either. She actually put on weight the first four weeks because, to her credit, she gave up smoking. Then there was a turning point.

I noticed her sweating with effort as she concentrated on the exercises—and Louise and I noticed her figure changing week by week at our weekly weigh- and measure-ins despite the fact that she was losing hardly any weight.

Kay, 49, says, "I began to feel more confident; it was an upward spiral – the more I saw my figure change for the better, the more I was determined to do the exercise. And, as my body improved, so did my self-image and confidence. It's a whole body thing—I used to walk along slowly; now I bounce along! And I feel more supple and lively. With more confidence, the upsets of divorce, and being laid off began to seem less threatening, and I could see possibilities for me. I realized I could make things happen. I've signed up for swimming lessons, and started training for a new career as a masseuse. I'm changing my life for the better, and I feel great!"

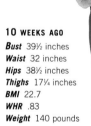

KAY 10 WEEKS AGO

Kay was, in her own words, "locked in a time warp," with her hair and makeup. She was badly in need of advice on dressing for her shape and on updating her wardrobe.

10 WEEKS AGO

Bust 39½ inches
Waist 32 inches
Hips 38½ inches
Thighs 17¼ inches
BMI 22.7
WHR .83
Weight 140 pounds

KAY NOW

Bust 39 inches
Waist 29¼ inches
Hips 37 inches
Thighs 18½ inches
BMI 22.4
WHR .79
Weight 138 pounds